The Caregiver

at

Geriatrics

MARTIN STERLING

Table of contents

Introduction — 15
- The essential role of the geriatric caregiver — 16
- The challenges of an ageing population — 17
- Objectives and structure of the book — 19

Chapter 1: Understanding geriatrics — 23

Physiological aging — 24
- Anatomical and physiological changes — 24
- Impact on organic systems — 28
- The concept of frailty in the elderly — 34

Pathological aging — 39
- The most common chronic diseases — 39
- Comorbidities and polypathologies — 45
- Differences between normal and pathological aging — 51

Psychological aspects of aging — 56
- Psychological adaptation in old age — 56

- Depression and mood disorders ... 62
- Importance of social and family support ... 68

Ethics and Deontology in Geriatrics ... 72
- Respect for dignity and autonomy ... 72
- Informed consent and patient rights ... 76
- Confidentiality and professional secrecy ... 81

Chapter 2: The role of the geriatric caregiver ... 87

Skills and Qualifications ... 88
- Basic medical knowledge ... 88
- Relational and communication skills ... 94
- Stress management and resilience ... 98

Responsibilities and role limits ... 102
- Authorized activities and delegated acts ... 102
- Collaboration with the care team ... 106
- Legal and professional liability ... 113

Relations with families and friends ... 118
- Empathetic communication ... 118
- Managing expectations and emotions ... 122
- Supporting care decisions ... 126

Chapter 3: Basic geriatric care — 133

Hygiene and Patient Comfort — 134
- Adapted grooming techniques — 134
- Skin care and pressure sore prevention — 139
- Installation and refurbishment of healthcare bed — 145

Nutrition and hydration — 152
- Specific nutritional requirements — 152
- Help with meals — 157
- Monitoring intake and swallowing disorders — 163

Mobilization and Travel — 168
- Safe handling techniques — 168
- Use of technical aids (walkers, wheelchairs) — 172
- Preventing falls and maintaining independence — 181

Urinary and faecal elimination — 186
- Assistance with natural needs — 186
- Incontinence management — 191
- Diuresis and stool monitoring — 196

Rest and Sleep — 200
- The importance of sleep-wake rhythms — 200

- Creating a restful environment — 206
- Detection of sleep disorders — 211

Chapter 4: Management of common pathologies — 217

Neurodegenerative diseases — 218

- Alzheimer's disease: signs and support — 218
- Dementia: types and non-drug approaches — 223
- Communication with disoriented patients — 231

Cardiovascular disorders — 236

- Heart failure: monitoring and warning signs — 236
- Hypertension: preventive measures — 242
- Stroke: post-stroke management — 248

Respiratory conditions — 255

- Chronic obstructive pulmonary disease (COPD) — 255
- Pneumonia: prevention and care — 262
- Use of oxygen therapy — 269

Musculoskeletal disorders — 274

- Osteoarthritis and rheumatism: pain management ... 274
- Osteoporosis: preventing fractures ... 277
- Mobilization assistance with respect for limitations ... 281

Diabetes in the Elderly ... 288
- Blood glucose monitoring ... 288
- Signs of hypo- and hyperglycemia ... 293
- Adapted diet ... 299

Chapter 5: Emergency situations and first-aid procedures ... 305

Recognizing emergency signs ... 306
- Respiratory distress ... 306
- Cardiorespiratory arrest ... 313
- Falls and injuries ... 319

First aid and emergency procedures ... 325
- Cardiopulmonary resuscitation (CPR) ... 325
- Lateral safety position (PLS) ... 330
- Using the automated external defibrillator (AED) ... 334

Alert and Reporting Procedures ... 340
- Rapid communication with the medical team ... 340
- Incident documentation ... 345

- Participation in post-incident debriefings   350

Chapter 6: Palliative and end-of-life care   355

Principles of Palliative Care   356

- Pain and symptom relief   356
- Quality of life and respect for patients' wishes   360
- Holistic approach: physical, psychological, social and spiritual   365

Accompanying patients at the end of life   370

- Presence and attentive listening   370
- Managing end-of-life events   374
- Respect for rituals and beliefs   380

Family support   384

- Communication on the evolution of the patient's condition   384
- Help with administrative formalities   390
- Presence in the final moments   394

Chapter 7: Technologies and Innovations in Geriatrics   401

E-health and telemedicine   402

- Using connected devices to monitor patients   402

- Advantages and limitations of remote monitoring — 406
- Impact on the role of the caregiver — 411

Technical Aids and Home Automation — 416

- Presentation of autonomy-enhancing tools (smart beds, motion sensors) — 416
- Training in the use of modern equipment — 421
- Integrating technology into daily care — 425

Mobile Applications and Tracking Software — 431

- Care management and patient records software — 431
- Applications for cognitive stimulation — 439

Assistance robots — 445

- Companion robots to combat isolation — 445
- Future prospects for robotics in geriatrics — 450

Chapter 8: Patient autonomy and health promotion — 457

Prevention of Age-Related Pathologies — 458

- Recommended vaccinations — 458
- Early detection of chronic diseases — 461

- Promoting a healthy lifestyle — 464

Social and therapeutic leisure activities — 466

- The importance of recreational activities for well-being — 466
- Organization of workshops and outings — 468
- Collaboration with animators and volunteers — 470

Chapter 9: Managing Cognitive and Behavioral Disorders — 473

A closer look at dementia — 474

- Differentiating between types of dementia — 474
- Symptoms and disease stages — 477
- Adapted intervention strategies — 481

Non-pharmacological approaches — 484

- Reminiscence therapies — 484
- Sensory and cognitive stimulation — 486
- Environmental design to reduce anxiety — 488

Managing psychological disorders — 491

- Recognizing depression and anxiety — 491
- Communication techniques to soothe the patient — 493

- Collaboration with psychologists and psychiatrists   496

Thanks   499

- **To all the dedicated professionals who work with the elderly every day.**   500

"Caring for our elders means honoring their lives and offering them the dignity they deserve at the end of their lives."

Introduction

- **The essential role of the geriatric caregiver**

In today's medical landscape, marked by an increasingly aging population, the geriatric caregiver occupies a central and irreplaceable position. Their mission goes far beyond technical care to encompass a global approach to the elderly person, integrating physical, psychological and social dimensions.

On a day-to-day basis, the caregiver is the first point of contact for elderly patients. They establish a fundamental relationship of trust, based on listening, respect and benevolence. This proximity enables them to perceive the slightest changes in the patient's state of health, whether somatic or emotional. For example, he can detect early signs of dehydration, unexpressed pain or emerging cognitive disorders, enabling rapid and appropriate intervention.

It also plays a preventive role. By helping patients with everyday tasks, they help prevent complications associated with immobility or dependency, such as bedsores, urinary tract infections or falls. They ensure that patients maintain the highest possible level of autonomy, stimulating them and encouraging them to take an active part in their care. This approach promotes not only physical well-being, but also the patient's self-esteem and quality of life.

Geriatric caregivers must have a sound knowledge of pathologies specific to old age, such as dementia, Parkinson's disease or heart failure. They need to understand the particularities of physiological aging, so they can adapt their interventions accordingly. For example, they will know that an elderly patient's skin is more fragile, requiring delicate grooming to avoid skin lesions.

On a relational level, they play a key role in providing psychological support to patients. Elderly people may experience anxiety, loneliness or depression in the face of loss of autonomy or illness. The caregiver is there to provide a reassuring presence, to listen without judgment, and to offer comfort. They also help maintain social ties, by encouraging participation in group activities or facilitating contact with family.

As part of a multidisciplinary team, the caregiver is an essential link in the chain. They work closely with nurses, doctors, physiotherapists and other healthcare professionals. They take part in oral and written communications, sharing their valuable observations which contribute to clinical decision-making. Their in-depth knowledge of the patient is an asset when it comes to tailoring personalized care plans.

Ethics play an important role in her practice. Respecting the patient's dignity, privacy and rights is at the heart of his concerns. He must be attentive to the elderly person's consent, even when the latter is cognitively impaired. They are also confronted with delicate situations, such as refusal of care or advance directives, requiring in-depth ethical reflection and appropriate communication.

Finally, the geriatric caregiver is faced with major emotional challenges, particularly at the end of life. They have to manage their own emotions, while offering quality support to patients and their families. This requires a high degree of professional maturity, resilience and personal commitment.

- **The challenges of an ageing population**

The XXIe century is marked by a major demographic transformation: the accelerated aging of the world's population. This development poses significant challenges to healthcare systems, social structures and, in particular, to professionals engaged in geriatric care, such as caregivers. Understanding these challenges is essential if we are to adapt practices and respond effectively to the growing needs of the elderly.

The aging of the population is the result of a combination of factors, including longer life expectancy thanks to medical advances and falling birth rates. According to demographic projections, the proportion of people aged 65 and over will continue to rise, bringing about a profound change in the age structure of society. This demographic transition is generating increased demand for long-term care, chronic disease prevention and support for activities of daily living.

In medical terms, ageing is accompanied by a higher prevalence of chronic pathologies such as cardiovascular disease, diabetes, neurodegenerative disorders such as Alzheimer's, and musculoskeletal disorders. The elderly often present complex co-morbidities, making therapeutic management more delicate. Caregivers therefore need to acquire in-depth expertise in recognizing atypical clinical signs, which are often masked or attenuated in geriatric patients.

Moreover, polymedication is common among the elderly, increasing the risk of adverse effects and drug interactions. Caregivers play a crucial role in monitoring medication compliance, detecting side effects and communicating with the multidisciplinary team to adjust treatments if necessary.

The challenges are not just medical. Aging is often accompanied by functional and cognitive losses, impacting on an individual's autonomy. Frailty, a geriatric syndrome characterized by a decline in physiological reserves, increases vulnerability to minor stresses and predisposes to unfavorable outcomes such as falls, repeated hospitalizations and increased dependency. Caregivers need to be trained in preventive approaches, focused on maintaining autonomy and functional rehabilitation.

In psychosocial terms, isolation and loneliness are major problems. The social network of the elderly can become restricted due to the death of loved ones, reduced mobility or social withdrawal linked to sensory or cognitive disorders. Caregivers are often at the forefront of this process, offering not only physical care but also empathic presence and moral support.

The economic stakes are also significant. The financing of geriatric care accounts for a growing share of healthcare expenditure. Care structures must adapt to offer efficient services while keeping costs under control. This means optimizing resources, increasing coordination between the various players in the healthcare system, and enhancing the role of caregivers as key elements in the care chain.

The ethical dimension cannot be ignored. Caregivers are faced with complex situations involving respect for autonomy, informed consent, management of advance directives and care of patients at the end of life. They must navigate between professional obligations, the expectations of patients and their families, and institutional constraints.

Moreover, the aging of the population highlights health disparities. Socio-economic inequalities influence access to care, quality of care and health outcomes among the elderly. Caregivers need to be sensitive to these issues to promote equity and tailor their interventions to the specific needs of each patient.

Finally, technological advances offer opportunities, but also pose challenges. The integration of telemedicine, connected devices and artificial intelligence into geriatric care requires appropriate training for healthcare professionals. For example, caregivers need to familiarize themselves with these tools to improve the quality of care, while ensuring respect for confidentiality and ethics.

- **Objectives and structure of the book**

This book has been designed to support and enhance the role of the geriatric caregiver, a profession at the heart of today's public health challenges. Faced with an aging demographic and increasingly complex needs of the elderly, it is essential to provide professionals with concrete tools and an in-depth understanding of their practice. The objectives of this book are manifold, and aim to provide a comprehensive, practical and inspiring resource for caregivers, whether students, novices or experienced.

The primary aim is to **provide a comprehensive and detailed guide** covering all aspects of the geriatric caregiver profession. This includes not only medical knowledge and care techniques, but also the interpersonal, ethical and organizational skills needed to excel in this field. By consolidating this information in an accessible format, we aim to facilitate learning and ongoing professional development.

Secondly, we aim to **reflect the day-to-day reality of the geriatric ward**, going beyond theories to address the concrete situations caregivers face. Through practical examples, case studies and testimonials, we seek to illustrate the challenges and rewards inherent in this profession. This immersive approach aims to prepare readers for complex situations and give them the tools to deal with them competently and confidently.

Another key objective is **to promote a humanistic, patient-centred approach**, emphasizing the dignity, autonomy and well-being of the elderly. We aim to raise caregivers' awareness of the importance of empathetic communication, respect for cultural diversity and the specific needs of each individual. By developing these aspects, the book encourages a care practice that is both professional and profoundly human.

In addition, we aim to **stimulate** caregivers' **ethical and professional reflection**. The situations encountered in geriatrics are often complex and require informed decision-making. By addressing ethical dilemmas, patient rights and legal obligations, we aim to guide professionals in a practice that conforms to the highest ethical standards.

Finally, the book aims to **prepare caregivers for future developments** in their profession, with chapters on technological innovations, geriatric care research and demographic perspectives. It encourages a proactive attitude to change, stressing the importance of ongoing training and adaptation to new practices.

The book's structure is designed to offer a logical and coherent progression, enabling readers to build up their knowledge in a fluid way. The book is divided into several main sections, each dealing with key themes in the geriatric caregiver profession.

The first part lays the **theoretical foundations**, exploring the understanding of aging, whether physiological, pathological or psychological. This section provides the essential foundations for understanding the specificities of elderly patients and adapting care accordingly.

The second part is dedicated to the **role of the caregiver**, detailing the skills required, responsibilities and limitations of the profession. It emphasizes multidisciplinary teamwork and communication with families, crucial elements in holistic care.

The third section covers **basic care and the management of common pathologies**, offering detailed protocols and practical advice for day-to-day interventions. This section aims to reinforce technical skills and promote best practice in care.

The fourth part focuses on **communication and the helping relationship**, recognizing the importance of the human aspect in geriatric care. It explores therapeutic communication techniques, management of behavioral problems and psychological support for patients and their families.

The fifth part deals with **special situations**, such as medical emergencies, palliative care and end-of-life support. It offers guidelines for acting effectively and compassionately in often difficult contexts.

Subsequent sections integrate **contemporary and innovative themes**, such as the use of technology in geriatrics, the consideration of cultural diversity, legal and ethical aspects, as well as research and evidence-based practices. These sections aim to broaden the perspective of caregivers and prepare them for the future challenges of their profession.

Finally, the book concludes **with testimonials, case studies and appendices**, providing additional resources to deepen knowledge and draw on the experience of colleagues.

Chapter 1

Understanding geriatrics

Physiological aging

- Anatomical and physiological changes

Aging is a natural process that brings about a series of progressive changes within the body, affecting both the anatomical structure and the physiological functioning of different systems. Understanding these changes is essential for the geriatric caregiver, as they influence how care must be adapted to meet the specific needs of the elderly.

Integumentary system

As we age, our skin undergoes significant transformations. It becomes thinner and less elastic due to reduced production of collagen and elastin in the dermis. The loss of subcutaneous adipose tissue reduces protection against trauma and temperature variations, making the skin more vulnerable to injury, ulceration and infection. The sebaceous and sweat glands are less active, leading to increased skin dryness and a reduced ability to regulate body temperature. In addition, the reduced number of melanocytes affects skin pigmentation, making it more sensitive to ultraviolet rays and predisposed to precancerous and cancerous lesions.

Musculoskeletal system

The musculoskeletal system is also affected by aging. Muscle mass gradually diminishes, a phenomenon known as sarcopenia, leading to a reduction in muscular strength and endurance. This loss of muscle is often associated with reduced physical activity and metabolic changes. Bones become more fragile due to reduced bone mineral density, increasing the risk of osteoporosis and fractures, particularly of the hip, wrist and vertebrae. Joints undergo degeneration of articular cartilage and changes in synovial fluid, which can lead to osteoarthritis, characterized by pain, stiffness and restricted movement.

Cardiovascular system

As the cardiovascular system ages, arterial walls become progressively stiffer as collagen builds up and elastic fibers lose their elasticity, a process known as arteriosclerosis. This arterial rigidity contributes to a rise in systolic blood pressure and an increased load on the heart. Myocardium can thicken, particularly in the left ventricle, reducing the heart's ability to fill efficiently. Maximum heart rate decreases, and the heart's response to beta-adrenergic stimuli is attenuated, which can limit exercise tolerance. Changes in the cardiac conduction system increase the risk of arrhythmias.

Respiratory system

The lungs lose elasticity due to changes in connective tissue, reducing total lung capacity. The rigidity of the rib cage increases due to calcification of the costal cartilages and reduced strength of respiratory muscles such as the diaphragm and intercostal muscles. These changes lead to a reduction in tidal volume and vital capacity, and an increase in residual volume. The function of epithelial cilia in the airways is impaired, reducing the efficiency of mucociliary clearance and increasing the risk of respiratory infections.

Gastrointestinal system

Aging also affects the digestive system. Saliva secretion may decrease, leading to xerostomia (dry mouth) which can affect chewing and swallowing. Esophageal motility is reduced, increasing the risk of dysphagia and gastro-esophageal reflux. Gastric acid secretion may be reduced, affecting protein digestion and the absorption of certain vitamins and minerals, such as vitamin B12, iron and calcium. Intestinal motility slows down, which can lead to chronic constipation. Liver function is generally preserved, but the hepatic metabolism of certain drugs may be impaired.

Renal and urinary system

The kidneys undergo a reduction in renal mass and a progressive loss of functional nephrons, which reduces glomerular filtration rate. This affects the kidney's ability to concentrate urine and excrete metabolic waste products, increasing the risk of hydro-electrolytic imbalances and accumulation of toxic substances. The ability to regulate acid-base balance is also reduced. In men, benign prostatic hypertrophy is common and can cause obstructive symptoms of the lower urinary tract, such as difficulty in initiating micturition, reduced urine flow and frequent nocturnal urination (nocturia). In women, relaxation of the pelvic floor muscles can lead to stress urinary incontinence.

Nervous system

The central nervous system undergoes mild cerebral atrophy due to neuronal loss and reduced neuron size. Nerve conduction is slowed due to degeneration of the myelin sheath, affecting reflexes and reaction time. These changes can lead to alterations in cognitive functions, including memory, attention and speed of information processing. However, brain plasticity can often partially compensate for these losses. The autonomic nervous system is also affected, with a reduction in the baroreflex response, which can lead to orthostatic hypotension and an increased risk of falls.

Direction

Sensory organs undergo changes that can alter perception. Vision is affected by presbyopia, a reduction in lens accommodation that makes close-up vision difficult. Cataracts, an opacification of the crystalline lens, and age-related macular degeneration can reduce visual acuity. Hearing diminishes due to presbycusis, a progressive loss of hair cells in the inner ear, particularly affecting high frequencies and complicating speech comprehension in noisy environments. Taste and smell are altered due to the loss of sensory receptors, which can diminish appetite and affect nutrition. Touch is less sensitive due to a reduction in the number of tactile receptors, affecting perception of pain, temperature and pressure.

Endocrine system

The endocrine system undergoes significant hormonal changes. Production of certain hormones declines, such as growth hormone, DHEA (dehydroepiandrosterone) and sex hormones (estrogen in women after menopause, testosterone in men). These changes can affect body composition, favoring an increase in fat mass and a decrease in lean mass. Insulin sensitivity may be reduced, increasing the risk of type 2 diabetes. Thyroid function is generally stable, but a slight decrease in thyroxine production may occur, slowing basal metabolism.

Immune system

Immune aging, or immunosenescence, is characterized by a reduction in the production and function of T and B lymphocytes. This alteration in cellular and humoral immunity reduces the body's ability to fight infections and respond effectively to vaccinations. Elderly people are therefore more likely to develop serious infections and have a less robust vaccine response. In addition, chronic low-grade systemic inflammation, known as "inflammaging", is often present, contributing to the development of chronic age-related diseases such as atherosclerosis, arthritis and Alzheimer's disease.

Implications for geriatric care

These anatomical and physiological changes have a direct impact on the care of elderly patients. Caregivers must adapt their interventions to take account of the increased fragility of the skin, using gentle mobilization techniques to prevent skin lesions and pressure sores. Monitoring nutrition and hydration is essential to prevent malnutrition and dehydration, taking into account changes in taste, smell and digestion.

Communication with patients may require adjustments, such as speaking distinctly and face-to-face to compensate for hearing deficits, or using visual aids in the case of vision impairment. Falls prevention is a priority, involving regular assessment of balance, muscle strength and environment to eliminate obstacles and risks.

Managing polymedication is another crucial aspect, as changes in pharmacokinetics and pharmacodynamics in the elderly increase the risk of adverse drug reactions. The caregiver must be vigilant in monitoring medication compliance, signs of overdose or drug interactions, and report any abnormalities to the nursing or medical team.

Finally, understanding cognitive and sensory changes enables the caregiver to adapt his or her approach, demonstrating patience, respect and empathy. It is important to stimulate the patient's remaining abilities, promote autonomy and maintain an active social life to preserve quality of life.

- Impact on organic systems

The aging process brings with it a series of anatomical and physiological changes that affect all the organic systems of the human body. These changes have a significant impact on the body's overall functioning, altering the ability of the elderly to maintain homeostasis and respond to physiological stresses. For the geriatric caregiver, it is essential to understand these impacts in order to adapt care and prevent associated complications.

Cardiovascular system

Aging of the cardiovascular system results in a reduction in the elasticity of blood vessels, particularly arteries, due to the loss of elastic fibers and the accumulation of collagen. This arterial stiffness increases peripheral resistance, leading to a rise in systolic blood pressure. The heart, for its part, undergoes moderate left ventricular hypertrophy in response to this increased workload. Myocardial relaxation capacity is reduced, affecting diastolic filling. These changes can lead to diastolic heart failure, where the heart is unable to fill adequately.

In addition, the cardiac conduction system is subject to fibrosis and lipid deposits, increasing the risk of arrhythmias such as atrial fibrillation. The baroreflex response is impaired, which can lead to orthostatic hypotension, increasing the risk of falls. The heart's ability to increase cardiac output during exercise is also diminished, limiting exercise tolerance and making the elderly more vulnerable to episodes of myocardial ischemia.

Respiratory system

Changes in the respiratory system affect the efficiency of gas exchange. Loss of pulmonary elasticity and increased ribcage rigidity reduce vital capacity and increase residual volume. Decreased strength of the respiratory muscles, including the diaphragm, compromises the ability to ventilate the lungs efficiently. Alveoli may dilate and their walls thin, reducing the exchange surface for oxygen and carbon dioxide.

These changes increase susceptibility to hypoxemia, particularly in the event of infection or heart failure. Mucociliary clearance is less efficient, due to the reduced number and activity of epithelial cilia, which favours the accumulation of secretions and the risk of respiratory infections such as pneumonia. Coughing and sneezing reflexes are also weakened, reducing the ability to expel pathogens or foreign bodies.

Immune system

Immunosenescence significantly affects immune function. The production of naive T lymphocytes decreases due to thymic involution, reducing the diversity of the cellular immune response. B lymphocytes show a reduced capacity to produce effective antibodies, affecting humoral immunity. This immune alteration makes the elderly more susceptible to infections, including opportunistic infections, and reduces the efficacy of vaccinations.

In addition, a state of chronic low-grade inflammation ("inflammaging") contributes to the development of chronic inflammatory diseases, such as atherosclerosis, type 2 diabetes and neurodegenerative diseases. Increased pro-inflammatory cytokines can also aggravate the symptoms of pre-existing diseases and affect recovery from acute illness.

Neurological system

Impacts on the central nervous system include a reduction in overall brain volume, particularly in the cortical and hippocampal regions associated with memory and cognition. Neuronal loss and reduced synapses affect the transmission of nerve signals, leading to a slowdown in cognitive functions such as working memory, information processing speed and learning capacity.

Mild neurocognitive disorders can progress to dementia, of which Alzheimer's disease is the most common form. Changes in the dopaminergic system can affect motor skills, leading to Parkinsonian syndromes. The peripheral nervous system is also affected, with reduced proprioceptive and tactile sensitivity, increasing the risk of injuries and falls.

Endocrine and metabolic systems

Hormonal changes influence metabolism and energy regulation. Reduced secretion of growth hormone and DHEA contributes to decreased muscle mass and increased body fat. Insulin resistance increases, predisposing to type 2 diabetes. Fluctuations in thyroid hormones can affect basal metabolism, leading to increased fatigue and cold intolerance.

In women, the menopause leads to a drop in estrogen, increasing the risk of osteoporosis and cardiovascular disease. In men, the gradual decline in testosterone can affect bone density, muscle mass and sexual function. These hormonal changes also have a psychological impact, contributing to depression and anxiety.

Renal and urinary system

Reduced glomerular filtration rate affects the kidneys' ability to eliminate metabolic waste and concentrate urine. This decrease in renal function increases the risk of drug and toxin accumulation, necessitating dosage adjustments and close monitoring of drug therapy. The ability to regulate fluid and electrolyte balance is compromised, making the elderly more susceptible to sodium, potassium and water imbalances, which can lead to dehydration or edema.

Structural changes in the urinary system, such as reduced bladder muscle tone and prostatic hypertrophy in men, lead to micturition disorders. Urinary incontinence is common, affecting quality of life and increasing the risk of urinary tract infections. Caregivers need to be alert to these problems, so they can implement preventive measures and appropriate interventions.

Digestive and nutritional systems

Impacts on the digestive system include reduced appetite due to sensory changes (altered taste and smell), mastication disorders linked to dental problems, and early satiety caused by slowed gastric emptying. These factors can lead to protein-energy malnutrition, further weakening the immune system and delaying wound healing.

Reduced intestinal absorption of certain vitamins and minerals, such as vitamin B12, iron and calcium, can lead to anemia and aggravate osteoporosis. Chronic constipation is common, due to slowed intestinal transit and reduced water and fiber intake. Particular attention must be paid to nutritional assessment and the implementation of appropriate diets.

Musculoskeletal system

Sarcopenia, characterized by loss of muscle mass and strength, reduces mobility and increases the risk of falls and fractures. Osteoporosis weakens bones, making fractures more likely even after minor trauma. Joint pain linked to osteoarthritis limits physical activity, creating a vicious circle of muscular deconditioning and loss of autonomy.

Impacts on the musculoskeletal system also affect posture and balance. Dorsal kyphosis due to vertebral compression can alter the center of gravity, increasing the risk of imbalance. Caregivers should encourage adapted physical exercise, physiotherapy and the use of mobility aids to maintain motor function.

Sensory systems

Reduced visual acuity due to presbyopia, cataracts or macular degeneration affects the ability to carry out daily activities and increases the risk of accidents in the home. Hearing loss, particularly of high frequencies, hampers communication, leading to social isolation and potentially dangerous misunderstandings (e.g. not hearing alarms).

Impaired taste and smell can lead to reduced food intake and accidental ingestion of harmful substances. Decreased tactile sensitivity affects the perception of pain, temperature and pressure, delaying the detection of wounds, burns or pressure areas likely to develop pressure sores.

Integumentary system

Fragile, less elastic skin is more prone to tears, pressure ulcers and infections. Reduced melanin production increases sensitivity to UV rays, raising the risk of skin cancers. Reduced cutaneous vascularization slows wound healing. Less active sweat glands affect thermoregulation, making the elderly more vulnerable to hypo- and hyperthermia.

Implications for overall management

The combined impact on body systems creates a situation of multidimensional fragility. Elderly people have reduced physiological reserves, which means their ability to respond to stress, whether physical (infection, injury) or psychological (stress, bereavement), is limited. Acute illness can rapidly decompensate underlying chronic conditions, requiring careful monitoring.

The complexity of co-morbidities and drug interactions demands an interdisciplinary approach. The caregiver plays a central role in detecting early signs of deterioration, promoting autonomy and coordinating care. It is essential to personalize interventions, taking into account the patient's residual abilities, preferences and socio-familial environment.

Communication with patients must be adapted to sensory deficits, using visual aids, ensuring a calm environment and confirming understanding of information. Psychological support is crucial to prevent depression, anxiety and social isolation. Cognitive and social stimulation activities help maintain brain function and quality of life.

Prevention is a major focus, including vaccination, promotion of physical exercise, adequate nutrition, prevention of falls and monitoring for signs of infection or decompensation. Educating patients and families about the impact of aging and preventive measures enhances the effectiveness of interventions.

Ethical considerations are also essential. Questions relating to consent, autonomous decision-making and advance directives must be approached with tact and respect. The caregiver must take care to preserve the patient's dignity, promote self-determination and support his or her rights.

- The concept of frailty in the elderly

The concept of frailty in the elderly is fundamental to geriatrics, as it characterizes a state of increased vulnerability to stress, whether medical, social or environmental. Frailty is not simply an inevitable consequence of aging, but a distinct clinical syndrome resulting from the body's diminishing physiological and functional reserves. Understanding this concept is essential for the geriatric caregiver, as it directly influences the care and interventions needed to preserve the health and autonomy of the elderly.

Definition and characteristics of fragility

Frailty is defined as a state of reduced reserve capacity in the body, which limits resistance to minor stress factors. This condition results from the complex interaction between biological aging processes, chronic diseases and psychosocial factors. Frail people have a diminished capacity to maintain homeostasis, which exposes them to an increased risk of adverse events such as falls, hospitalization, institutionalization and mortality.

Key features of fragility include:

- **Involuntary weight loss**: often linked to reduced muscle mass (sarcopenia) and poor nutrition.
- **Fatigue or exhaustion**: persistent feeling of tiredness that affects daily activities.

- **Muscular weakness**: measured by reduced grip strength or other physical performance tests.
- **Slow gait**: indicative of mobility and balance problems.
- **Low level of physical activity**: reduced participation in usual activities, which can worsen muscle loss and endurance.

These criteria, known as Fried's frailty phenotype, identify frail individuals when at least three of these signs are present. The presence of one or two criteria indicates a state of pre-fragility, which represents an intermediate phase where preventive interventions can be particularly effective.

Pathophysiology of frailty

Fragility is the result of an accumulation of deficits across various physiological systems, creating a synergistic effect that exceeds the sum of individual deficits. Underlying mechanisms include:

- **Sarcopenia**: the progressive loss of muscle mass and strength due to hormonal and metabolic changes and reduced physical activity.
- **Chronic inflammation**: a state of low-grade inflammation, often referred to as "inflammaging", which contributes to tissue degradation and organ dysfunction.
- **Mitochondrial dysfunction**: affecting cellular energy production, reducing the body's ability to meet increased metabolic needs.
- **Oxidative stress**: the accumulation of free radicals damages cells and tissues, accelerating biological aging.
- **Neuroendocrine alterations**: changes in the regulation of anabolic and catabolic hormones, impacting tissue regeneration and stress response.

These interconnected processes lead to an overall reduction in functional reserves, making the individual more likely to fall into a state of decompensation in the event of minor stress.

Clinical consequences of frailty

Fragility has major clinical implications:

- **Increased risk of falls**: due to muscle weakness, impaired balance and slower reflexes.
- **Accelerated functional decline**: rapid loss of autonomy in activities of daily living (ADL) and instrumental activities of daily living (IADL).
- **Frequent hospitalizations**: frail people are more likely to be hospitalized for acute problems, and are at greater risk of nosocomial complications.
- **Prolonged recovery**: after illness or surgery, recovery time is often longer, with an increased risk of complications.
- **Increased mortality**: frailty is an independent predictor of short- and long-term mortality.

Fragility assessment

Assessing frailty is essential to identifying people at risk and implementing appropriate interventions. Several tools are used:

- **Fried phenotype**: based on the five criteria mentioned above.
- **Rockwood frailty index**: quantifies frailty in terms of the number of deficits accumulated in various clinical, functional and psychosocial parameters.
- **The Short Physical Performance Battery (SPPB)**: assesses physical performance through tests of walking, balance and muscular strength.
- **The FRAIL questionnaire**: a simple tool based on five questions relating to fatigue, resistance, ambulation, illness and weight loss.

A comprehensive assessment should also include a review of cognitive function, nutritional status, mental health and social support.

Interventions to prevent and manage frailty

As frailty is a potentially reversible condition, especially at an early stage, interventions must be multidisciplinary:

- **Physical exercise**: resistance training programs (weight training), balance exercises and aerobic activities have been shown to improve muscle strength, mobility and reduce the risk of falls.
- **Nutrition**: a diet rich in protein, sufficient calories, and essential micronutrients (vitamins D, B12, calcium) is crucial to supporting muscle mass and bone health.
- **Eliminate polymedication**: regularly review medication regimens to avoid harmful interactions and undesirable effects that can aggravate frailty.
- **Psychosocial support**: encourage social interaction, participate in community activities, and treat depression or anxiety, which can contribute to isolation and reduced activity.
- **Functional rehabilitation**: physiotherapy and occupational therapy interventions to improve functional abilities and autonomy.
- **Falls prevention**: assessment and modification of the home environment to eliminate risks, use of appropriate technical aids.

The caregiver's role in managing frailty

The caregiver is in a privileged position to detect the first signs of frailty and intervene effectively:

- **Observation and reporting**: be alert to subtle changes in the patient's physical and mental state, such as loss of appetite, excessive fatigue, reduced mobility or interest in usual activities.
- **Promoting physical activity**: encouraging and assisting patients with simple exercises, adapted to their abilities, to maintain or improve muscle strength and balance.

- **Nutritional support**: ensuring that patients receive adequate nutrition, in collaboration with dieticians, and assisting with meals if necessary.
- **Education**: informing patients and their families about frailty, its consequences and ways to prevent or delay it.
- **Care coordination**: working closely with the multidisciplinary team to ensure coherent care adapted to the patient's specific needs.
- **Emotional support**: offering empathetic listening, helping to maintain morale and encourage social relations to combat isolation.

The importance of prevention

Preventing frailty is a major objective in geriatrics. It involves early action to maintain functional capacities and delay dependency:

- **Early detection**: identify people in a state of pre-fragility and intervene before the situation worsens.
- **Promoting a healthy lifestyle**: encouraging a balanced diet, regular physical activity and an active social life.
- **Vaccinations and infection prevention**: infections can have serious consequences in fragile people, so vaccination and hygiene measures are essential.
- **Proactive management of chronic diseases**: optimal control of existing pathologies reduces stress on the body and prevents worsening of frailty.

Ethical and social considerations

The management of frailty also raises ethical issues:

- **Respecting autonomy**: involving patients in decisions concerning their health and care, while respecting their preferences and values.
- **Informed consent**: ensuring that the patient understands the proposed interventions and their implications.
- **Equal access to care**: ensuring that all patients, regardless of their socio-economic situation, have access to the necessary interventions.
- **Support for caregivers**: families and loved ones play a crucial role; supporting them is essential for effective care.

Pathological aging

- The most common chronic diseases

The elderly are particularly exposed to a number of chronic illnesses that have a profound impact on their quality of life and independence. These often interconnected pathologies require comprehensive, personalized care. For the geriatric caregiver, in-depth knowledge of these illnesses is essential to provide appropriate care and prevent complications. Here's an overview of the most common chronic diseases affecting the elderly.

1. Cardiovascular disease

Cardiovascular disease is the leading cause of morbidity and mortality in the elderly. They include :

- **Arterial hypertension (AHT)**: Chronic elevation of blood pressure, often asymptomatic, increases the risk of stroke, myocardial infarction and kidney failure. The caregiver must regularly monitor blood pressure, be alert to clinical signs such as headaches and dizziness, and encourage compliance with hygienic and dietary measures.

- **Heart failure**: results from the heart's inability to pump enough blood to meet the body's needs. Symptoms include shortness of breath, fatigue, edema of the lower limbs and rapid weight gain. The caregiver plays a key role in monitoring symptoms, managing fluid and sodium intake, and ensuring compliance with treatment.
- **Coronary artery disease**: due to atherosclerosis of the coronary arteries, it can cause angina pectoris and myocardial infarction. Warning signs include chest pain, shortness of breath and palpitations. Prompt treatment is essential to limit damage to the heart.

2. Type 2 diabetes

Type 2 diabetes is characterized by chronic hyperglycemia due to insulin resistance. In the elderly, it may be asymptomatic or manifest as fatigue, polyuria, polydipsia and weight loss. Long-term complications include:

- **Macrovascular complications**: Increased risk of stroke, coronary heart disease and peripheral arterial disease.
- **Microvascular complications**: kidney damage (diabetic nephropathy), eye damage (retinopathy) and nerve damage (peripheral neuropathy).

The caregiver must monitor blood sugar levels, be alert to signs of hypoglycemia or hyperglycemia, and encourage a balanced diet and appropriate physical activity.

3. Chronic respiratory diseases

- **Chronic obstructive pulmonary disease (COPD)**: This disease is characterized by progressive, irreversible airway obstruction, often due to smoking. Symptoms include chronic cough, sputum production and dyspnea. The caregiver must help manage secretions, encourage respiratory physiotherapy and monitor for signs of exacerbation.

4. Osteoporosis

Osteoporosis is a disease characterized by a decrease in bone density, increasing the risk of fractures, particularly of the hip, spine and wrist. Risk factors include advanced age, female gender, menopause, calcium and vitamin D deficiency. The caregiver must:

- **Prevent falls**: Secure the environment, use mobility aids.
- **Encourage a diet rich in calcium and vitamin D.**
- **Encourage physical exercise**: weight-bearing activities to strengthen bones.

5. Neurodegenerative diseases

- **Alzheimer's disease and other dementias**: characterized by progressive deterioration of memory, cognitive functions and behavior. Symptoms include impaired memory, orientation, language and personality changes. The caregiver must:
    - **Adopt appropriate communication**: use simple sentences, be patient.
    - **Ensure patient safety**: Prevent wandering and domestic accidents.
    - **Support cognitive activities**: Stimulate memory and executive functions.
- **Parkinson's disease**: characterized by muscular rigidity, resting tremors and bradykinesia. Patients may also have balance and coordination problems. The caregiver must:
    - **Assisting mobility**: Use safe transfer techniques.
    - **Monitor swallowing**: Prevent false swallowing.
    - **Encourage adherence to treatment**: Monitor side effects of antiparkinsonian drugs.

6. Chronic renal failure

This pathology is due to a progressive deterioration in kidney function, leading to an accumulation of metabolic waste in the body. Symptoms may include fatigue, nausea, edema and hypertension. The caregiver must:

- **Monitor fluid intake**: Respect restrictions if prescribed.
- **Observe for signs of edema**: particularly around the ankles and eyelids.
- **Encourage a suitable diet**: low in sodium, potassium and phosphorus as recommended.

7. Sensory disorders

- **Presbycusis**: Age-related progressive loss of hearing, affecting high frequencies. The caregiver must:
    - **Communicate effectively**: Speak clearly, face-to-face, in a calm environment.
    - **Check the hearing aid**: Make sure it's working properly.
- **Presbyopia and other visual disorders**: reduced visual acuity, cataracts, macular degeneration. The caregiver must:
    - **Ensure a well-lit environment**.
    - **Help with the use of glasses or other devices**.

8. Psychiatric disorders

- **Depression**: Common in the elderly, it can be under-diagnosed. Symptoms include persistent sadness, loss of interest, sleep disturbances and fatigue. The caregiver must:
    - **Listening**: Encouraging the expression of feelings.
    - **Encourage social and physical activities**.

- ◦ **Report signs of depression to the medical team**.
- **Anxiety**: may manifest as agitation, insomnia, excessive worry. Empathic support is essential.

9. Osteoarticular diseases

- **Osteoarthritis**: Degenerative joint disease causing pain, stiffness and reduced mobility. It mainly affects the knees, hips and spine. The caregiver must:
  - ◦ **Help with mobilization**: Encourage gentle, adapted movements.
  - ◦ **Pain management**: Apply non-pharmacological measures such as heat.
  - ◦ **Facilitating daily activities**: Use technical aids if necessary.

10. Digestive disorders

- **Chronic constipation**: due to reduced intestinal motility, inadequate hydration, low-fiber diet. The caregiver must:
  - ◦ **Encourage hydration**: Encourage regular drinking.
  - ◦ **Promote a high-fiber diet**: fruit, vegetables, wholegrain cereals.
  - ◦ **Encourage physical activity**: Even a light walk can help.
- **Swallowing disorders (dysphagia)**: Increased risk of false routes. The caregiver must:
  - ◦ **Adapting food textures**: Blended foods, thickeners for liquids.
  - ◦ **Position the patient correctly during meals**: Sitting, head slightly tilted forward.
  - ◦ **Watch for signs of coughing or choking**.

11. Chronic infections

- **Urinary tract infections**: Common in the elderly, sometimes asymptomatic or manifesting as confusion or agitation. The caregiver must:
    - **Monitor urination habits**: frequency, pain, odour.
    - **Encourage good personal hygiene**.
    - **Promote adequate hydration**.
- **Respiratory infections**: the elderly are more vulnerable to influenza and pneumonia. The caregiver must:
    - **Encourage vaccination**: seasonal flu, pneumococcus.
    - **Promote hygiene measures**: washing hands, wearing masks if necessary.

12. Cancer

The risk of developing cancer increases with age. The most common cancers in the elderly include:

- **Lung cancer**: Linked to smoking, pollution. The caregiver must be alert to signs such as persistent cough, shortness of breath, hemoptysis.
- **Colon cancer**: warning signs such as changes in bowel habits, blood in the stool.
- **Breast and prostate cancer**: Monitoring abnormalities, encouraging screening.

The caregiver's role in chronic disease management

The caregiver is a key player in the management of chronic diseases in the elderly. Responsibilities include:

- **Clinical monitoring**: Observe and report changes in health status, signs of aggravation or complications.

- **Assistance with daily care**: Helping with activities of daily living while encouraging independence.
- **Promoting therapeutic compliance**: helping people to take their medication correctly, explaining the importance of taking it.
- **Patient and family education**: provide information on the disease, preventive measures and warning signs.
- **Psychological support**: listening, offering comfort, encouraging social participation.
- **Coordination with the healthcare team**: Communicate effectively with nurses, doctors and physiotherapists to ensure comprehensive care.

Prevention and health promotion

- **Balanced nutrition**: Encourage nutrition adapted to the patient's needs.
- **Regular physical activity**: Adapt exercises to the patient's abilities to maintain mobility and muscle strength.
- **Vaccinations**: Promoting protection against preventable infections.
- **Lifestyle**: advice on smoking cessation and alcohol moderation.

- Comorbidities and polypathologies

The term *comorbidity* refers to the simultaneous presence of several diseases or disorders in the same individual. In the elderly, the coexistence of multiple pathologies, known as *polypathology*, is a frequent phenomenon and represents a major challenge for geriatric care. Understanding the mechanisms, clinical implications and management strategies of co-morbidities is essential for the caregiver, who plays a crucial role in the care and well-being of polypathological patients.

1. Nature and prevalence of comorbidities in the elderly

With advancing age, individuals accumulate risk factors and organ damage that favor the development of various chronic diseases. Pathophysiological processes such as chronic inflammation, oxidative stress and weakened cellular repair systems contribute to the onset of multiple pathologies. For example, it is common for an elderly person to suffer simultaneously from cardiovascular disease, diabetes, osteoarthritis, kidney failure, cognitive impairment and other conditions.

Polypathology in the elderly is often associated with increased frailty, reduced autonomy and impaired quality of life. It complicates medical management due to interactions between diseases, treatment side-effects and the need to adapt interventions to the patient's capabilities.

2. Impact of co-morbidities on health and well-being

Comorbidities influence the health of the elderly in several ways:

- **Pathological interactions**: Diseases can aggravate each other. For example, poorly controlled diabetes can accelerate atherosclerosis, increasing the risk of cardiovascular disease. Heart failure can aggravate renal failure by reducing renal blood flow.

- **Therapeutic complexity**: The need to treat several diseases simultaneously leads to polymedication, increasing the risk of drug interactions, adverse effects and non-compliance. Side effects can be confused with disease symptoms, complicating diagnosis and treatment.

- **Reduced autonomy**: Co-morbidities can lead to a progressive loss of functional abilities, affecting activities of daily living (ADL) and instrumental activities of daily living (IADL). This leads to increased dependence on caregivers and family and friends.

- **Psychosocial impact**: Managing multiple illnesses can lead to stress, anxiety, depression and reduced quality of life. Social isolation can be exacerbated by physical limitations and frequent hospitalizations.

3. Challenges in managing polypathological patients

The care of polypathological elderly people presents several challenges:

- **Global assessment**: A holistic view of the patient is essential, taking into account all pathologies, functional, cognitive and nutritional abilities, as well as the patient's socio-familial environment.

- **Prioritizing care**: Determining treatment priorities according to the impact of diseases on quality of life and prognosis. Sometimes, it may be necessary to prioritize symptom control and comfort over the continuation of aggressive treatments.

- **Treatment adjustment**: Drug doses should be adjusted according to renal and hepatic function, and to the increased sensitivity to drugs in the elderly. Simplifying treatment regimens can improve compliance.

- **Preventing drug interactions**: Particular attention must be paid to drugs that are potentially inappropriate for the elderly, and to dangerous combinations.

- **Interprofessional communication**: Coordination between different healthcare professionals is crucial to ensure coherent care and avoid redundant or contradictory treatments.

4. Role of the caregiver in comorbidity management

The caregiver is strategically positioned to contribute effectively to the care of polypathological patients:

- **Observation and vigilance**: Monitor the clinical signs of various diseases, and be alert to changes in the patient's state of health, such as the appearance of new symptoms, worsening of existing symptoms, or undesirable effects of treatments.

- **Therapeutic compliance support**: Help patients to follow their treatment, respecting schedules, doses and conditions. Explain, if necessary, the importance of each medication and the consequences of non-adherence.

- **Health education**: informing patients and their families about the diseases present, measures to prevent complications, and warning signs requiring medical consultation.

- **Assistance with daily activities**: Helping the patient to carry out ADLs and IADLs, while encouraging the maintenance of autonomy wherever possible.

- **Prevent complications**: Participate in preventive measures, such as mobilization to avoid pressure sores, monitoring hydration and nutrition, preventing falls, following hygiene protocols to avoid infections.

- **Psychological support**: offering empathetic listening, helping patients to express their concerns, fears and frustrations related to the disease. Encourage social activities and relationships with family and friends.

5. The importance of care coordination

Polypathology requires a multidisciplinary approach. The caregiver must work closely with :

- **Nurses**: For clinical monitoring, treatment administration, dressing management and technical care.

- **Physicians**: To report observations, participate in overall geriatric assessments, understand therapeutic objectives.

- **Pharmacists**: For treatment review, prevention of drug interactions, drug education.

- **Physiotherapists and occupational therapists**: For functional rehabilitation, adaptation of the environment and promotion of autonomy.

- **Psychologists**: For emotional support, managing depression or anxiety.

- **Social workers**: to help set up home services, access financial aid and support family carers.

6. Strategies for improving quality of life in polypathological patients

- **Patient-centered approach**: Consider patient preferences, values and goals when planning care. Respect the patient's autonomy and right to make decisions.

- **Individualized care plan**: Adapt interventions to the patient's specific needs, taking into account his or her abilities and limitations.

- **Proactive symptom management**: Anticipating exacerbations of chronic diseases, implementing protocols for managing pain, dyspnea and anxiety.

- **Promoting physical activity**: Encouraging adapted exercise to maintain mobility and muscle strength and prevent deconditioning.

- **Nutritional support**: Ensure a balanced diet, adapted to the dietary restrictions associated with different pathologies (e.g. low-carb diet for diabetes, low-salt diet for hypertension).

- **Regular assessment of treatments**: Participate in medication reviews, report adverse effects, help adjust treatments in collaboration with the medical team.

7. Prevention of co-morbidities

Although certain comorbidities are inevitable with age, preventive measures can reduce their incidence or delay their onset:

- **Promoting a healthy lifestyle**: Encouraging smoking cessation, moderate alcohol consumption, a balanced diet and regular physical activity.

- **Vaccinations**: Encourage vaccination against influenza, pneumococcus and shingles to prevent infections that can decompensate chronic illnesses.

- **Early detection**: Participate in screening programs for cancer, osteoporosis and cognitive disorders.

- **Health education**: raising patients' awareness of modifiable risk factors, early signs of disease, and the importance of regular medical consultation.

8. Ethical and social considerations

Managing co-morbidities raises ethical issues:

- **Medication load**: Balancing the benefits and risks of treatments, avoiding over-treatment.

- **Quality of life vs. prolongation of life**: Discuss priorities with patient and family, respect advance directives.

- **Respecting autonomy**: Involve patients in decision-making, even in the presence of cognitive disorders, by adapting communication.

- **Caregiver support**: Recognize the burden on caregivers, offer them resources and respite.

9. Continuing education for caregivers

Faced with the complexity of comorbidities, it is essential that the caregiver :

- **Update your knowledge**: Keep abreast of developments in chronic disease management and new recommendations.

- **Develops specific skills**: pain management, communication with patients with cognitive disorders, use of technical aids.

- **Participate in multidisciplinary training**: To improve care coordination and understand the role of each professional.

- Differences between normal and pathological aging

Aging is a natural and inevitable process that affects all living beings. It is characterized by a series of physiological, biological and psychosocial changes that occur over time. However, it is essential to distinguish normal, or physiological, aging from pathological aging. This distinction is crucial for the geriatric caregiver, as it influences the way care is delivered and the interventions put in place to preserve the health and well-being of the elderly.

Normal (physiological) aging

Normal aging refers to the gradual, universal changes that occur with age, independent of disease or adverse environmental factors. These changes reflect the passage of time and do not necessarily hinder the individual's ability to lead an active, independent life. Here are some characteristics of normal aging:

- **Sensory changes**: A progressive decline in visual acuity (presbyopia), hearing (presbycusis) and taste is common. These changes can be compensated for by glasses, hearing aids or dietary adaptations.

- **Changes in body composition**: There is a reduction in muscle mass (sarcopenia) and a relative increase in fat mass. This can lead to reduced strength and endurance, but regular physical activity can mitigate these effects.

- **Skin changes**: Skin becomes thinner, less elastic and drier as a result of reduced collagen and elasticity. This is considered a normal part of skin aging.

- **Cardiovascular changes**: A slight increase in systolic blood pressure may occur due to increased arterial stiffness. However, this rise remains within normal limits for age and does not cause any symptoms.

- **Decreased lung capacity**: Maximum vital capacity decreases with age, but this does not generally affect daily activities unless intense physical effort is involved.

- **Renal and hepatic function**: There is a progressive reduction in renal and hepatic function, but these organs generally retain sufficient functional reserve to maintain homeostasis.

- **Cognitive changes**: Slower information processing and minor difficulties with short-term memory may occur. However, overall intellectual capacity and long-term memory remain intact.

- **Adaptation to stress**: Compensation mechanisms for physical or emotional stress are less effective, requiring a longer recovery period.

Pathological aging

Pathological aging, on the other hand, is characterized by diseases or disorders that are not an inevitable consequence of age, but occur more frequently in older people. These conditions go beyond the changes expected of normal aging, and result in significant impairment of health, function or quality of life. Here are just a few examples:

- **Neurodegenerative diseases**: Alzheimer's disease and other forms of dementia are not a normal part of aging. They manifest as a progressive deterioration of cognitive functions, affecting memory, language, judgment and behavior.

- **Cardiovascular disease**: Severe hypertension, heart failure, ischemic heart disease and stroke are the result of pathological processes such as atherosclerosis, not normal aging.

- **Type 2 diabetes**: Although the risk of diabetes increases with age, this disease is due to a combination of genetic and environmental factors, including lifestyle, and is not a direct consequence of aging.

- **Severe osteoporosis**: Excessive bone loss leading to pathological fractures is considered a disease, although bone density naturally decreases with age.

- **Disabling osteoarthritis**: While some joint degeneration is to be expected, osteoarthritis that causes chronic pain and functional disability is pathological.

- **Chronic renal failure**: A moderate reduction in renal function is normal, but renal failure requiring dialysis or leading to serious complications is pathological.

- **Depression and psychiatric disorders**: Major depression is not a normal consequence of aging, and requires appropriate management.

- **Cancers**: Although the risk of cancer increases with age, the development of malignant tumors is due to genetic mutations and environmental factors, not to the aging process itself.

Main differences between normal and pathological aging

1. **Nature of changes**: Normal aging involves gradual, predictable changes that do not significantly impair function or quality of life. Pathological aging is characterized by specific diseases that lead to clinical symptoms, suffering and reduced autonomy.

2. **Reversibility and prevention**: The changes of normal aging cannot be avoided, but their impact can be mitigated by a healthy lifestyle. The diseases of pathological aging can often be prevented, delayed or treated through medical interventions, primary and secondary prevention.

3. **Impact on function and autonomy**: In normal aging, individuals generally maintain good physical and cognitive function, enabling independent living. The

diseases of pathological aging can lead to dependence, incapacity and the need for long-term care.

4. **Need for medical intervention**: Normal aging does not require specific medical treatment, although some adaptations may be necessary. Pathological aging requires medical management, pharmacological treatments, surgical interventions or rehabilitation therapies.

5. **Individual variability**: Normal aging changes occur in all individuals, although their degree may vary. Pathological aging affects certain individuals, depending on genetic, environmental and lifestyle factors, and exposure to specific risks.

Implications for the geriatric caregiver

The distinction between normal and pathological aging has practical implications for the caregiver:

- **Accurate assessment**: The caregiver must be able to recognize signs that go beyond normal aging. For example, mild memory loss may be normal, but temporal or spatial disorientation requires medical attention.

- **Monitoring and reporting**: Being in close contact with the patient, the caregiver is well placed to detect subtle changes. They must report any suspicious changes in the patient's state of health to the nursing team.

- **Patient and family education**: It's important to inform patients and their families about the changes expected in normal aging, and to make them aware of the warning signs of pathological diseases.

- **Adapting care**: Understanding differences enables care to be adapted appropriately. For example, for a patient with age-related sarcopenia, the caregiver will encourage moderate physical exercise. In the case of a neurodegenerative disease, he or she will implement specific strategies to support memory and security.

- **Promoting prevention**: By knowing the risk factors for pathological diseases, the caregiver can promote healthy behaviors such as a balanced diet, physical activity, regular medical check-ups and vaccinations.

- **Psychological support**: Recognizing the difference between normal and pathological changes helps to address patient concerns, reduce age-related anxiety and provide appropriate support when illness is diagnosed.

Psychological aspects of aging

- Psychological adaptation in old age

Aging is a complex process that involves not only physical and biological changes, but also profound psychological transformations. Psychological adaptation in old age is a major issue for the well-being of the elderly, influencing their quality of life, autonomy and ability to cope with the challenges of old age. For the geriatric caregiver, understanding these psychological processes is essential to providing appropriate, empathetic and effective support.

Psychological transformations associated with aging

With advancing age, individuals are confronted with a series of changes that can affect their mental equilibrium:

1. **Life review and introspection**: Older people tend to take stock of their lives, revisiting memories, achievements, regrets and failures. This introspection can lead to a sense of accomplishment or, on the

contrary, to existential distress if they experience unresolved regrets.

2. **Changing social roles**: Retirement, the departure of children from the family home, the loss of a spouse or close friends can lead to a redefinition of social and family roles. This transition can lead to a sense of loss of purpose or identity.

3. **Facing up to finitude**: heightened awareness of mortality can lead to deep reflection on the meaning of life, existential anguish or, for some, a serene acceptance of the end of life.

4. **Loss of autonomy and body changes**: Physical limitations, chronic illness and changes in appearance can affect self-image and self-esteem, sometimes leading to frustration or shame.

5. **Reduced social network**: The death of loved ones, geographical distance from family and a shrinking circle of friends can lead to social isolation, a risk factor for mental health.

Psychic adaptation mechanisms

Faced with these changes, the elderly mobilize various coping mechanisms to maintain their psychological equilibrium:

1. **Resilience**: The ability to overcome adversity and adapt positively to difficult situations. Resilience can be enhanced by a strong support network, personal beliefs and effective coping strategies.

2. **Cognitive and emotional flexibility**: The ability to adjust thoughts and emotions in the face of new realities, adopting different perspectives and accepting what cannot be changed.

3. **Involvement in meaningful activities**: Participation in leisure, volunteer, cultural or spiritual activities that bring personal meaning and satisfaction.

4. **Social support**: Maintaining and developing relationships with family, friends and the community, offering emotional and practical support.

5. **Humor and derision**: Using humor to cope with difficulties, put problems into perspective and maintain a positive attitude.

6. **Spirituality and religion**: For some, faith and spiritual practices are a source of comfort, hope and meaning in the face of the challenges of old age.

Factors influencing psychological adaptation

Several factors can facilitate or hinder the psychological adaptation of the elderly:

- **Personality and individual traits**: Personality traits such as optimism, proactivity and self-confidence influence how a person deals with aging.

- **Mental health history**: People with a history of anxiety or depressive disorders may be more vulnerable to psychological difficulties in old age.

- **Life experiences**: Overcoming life's trials and tribulations can strengthen resilience, while unresolved traumas can resurface and affect psychological balance.

- **Family and social support**: A strong support network provides a buffer against stress and promotes better adaptation.

- **Level of education and socio-economic status**: Access to resources, information and care influences the ability to cope with the challenges of aging.

Psychological disorders common in the elderly

Despite their ability to adapt, some elderly people can develop mental disorders that require special attention:

1. **Depression**: Often under-diagnosed in the elderly, depression can manifest itself as persistent sadness, loss of interest in activities, sleep disorders, fatigue and suicidal thoughts. It can be confused with the symptoms of normal aging or the side effects of medication.

2. **Anxiety**: Anxiety disorders can be characterized by excessive worry, agitation and somatic complaints. Anxiety may be linked to concerns about health, safety or the future.

3. **Complicated mourning**: The loss of a spouse or loved one can lead to prolonged or pathological mourning, with depressive symptoms, disorientation and an inability to resume normal activities.

4. **Sleep disorders**: Insomnia and frequent waking at night can affect mood, cognition and physical health.

5. **Cognitive disorders**: Although dementias are neurodegenerative diseases, they have significant psychological repercussions, such as confusion, agitation and hallucinations.

The caregiver's role in psychological support

The caregiver plays an essential role in the psychological support of the elderly:

1. **Active, empathic listening**: providing an attentive presence, allowing patients to express their feelings and concerns without judgment.

2. **Observation of clinical signs**: Detect symptoms of depression, anxiety and confusion, and report them to the medical team for appropriate management.

3. **Cognitive and social stimulation**: Encourage participation in intellectual activities, memory games and discussions, to maintain cognitive function and prevent isolation.

4. **Promoting autonomy**: Valuing patients' remaining abilities, supporting them in activities they can still perform alone, boosting their self-esteem.

5. **Adapting communication**: Use clear language, simple sentences, rephrase if necessary, respect the patient's rhythm.

6. **Respecting habits and preferences**: Maintain the patient's routines as far as possible, respecting their choices, beliefs and values.

7. **Transition support**: Accompany the patient during important changes, such as admission to an institution or return home after hospitalization, by offering emotional support.

8. **Collaboration with families**: Involve family members in the care plan, keep them informed and support them in their role as caregivers.

Specific interventions to promote psychological adaptation

- **Non-pharmacological therapies**: Cognitive-behavioral therapies, reminiscence therapy, music therapy and art therapy can help improve mood, reduce anxiety and stimulate cognition.

- **Adapted physical activity**: Moderate physical exercise helps improve mood, sleep quality and overall physical health.

- **Stress management**: Relaxation techniques, deep breathing and meditation can be taught to reduce stress and anxiety.

- **Improving the environment**: Creating a safe, pleasant, sensory-stimulating environment, with temporal and spatial cues.

- **Pharmacological interventions**: In some cases, antidepressants, anxiolytics or other medications may be prescribed. The caregiver must monitor efficacy and side effects, and ensure compliance.

Prevention of mental disorders

Prevention is crucial:

- **Promoting well-being**: Encouraging healthy eating, regular sleep and pleasant activities.

- **Early detection**: Be alert to the first signs of psychological distress so you can intervene quickly.

- **Patient and family education**: provide information on normal aging, mental disorders and available resources.

- **Strengthening social support**: Facilitating contact with family, friends, support groups and community activities.

Ethical and cultural considerations

- **Respect for dignity**: treating each patient with respect, preserving his or her privacy and decision-making autonomy.

- **Informed consent**: Ensure that the patient understands the proposed interventions, and respect his or her choices, even in the event of disagreement, unless his or her safety is at stake.

- **Person-centered approach**: Personalize care according to the patient's needs, preferences and life history.

- **Cultural sensitivity**: Take into account the patient's beliefs, cultural values and religious practices when drawing up the care plan.

Training and professional development for caregivers

To be effective in psychological support :

- **Continuing education**: Keep abreast of advances in geriatric psychology and new therapeutic approaches.

- **Supervision and support**: Participate in supervision groups to share experiences and manage professional stress.

- **Ethical reflection**: Developing a reflection on ethical dilemmas, end-of-life issues and patients' rights.

- Depression and mood disorders

Depression and mood disorders in the elderly are major issues in geriatric medicine, often underestimated and inadequately managed. These psychological disorders have a considerable impact on the quality of life, autonomy and physical health of elderly patients. For the geriatric caregiver, it is essential to understand the clinical manifestations, risk factors, consequences and intervention strategies in order to provide appropriate and effective support.

Characteristics of depression in the elderly

Depression in the elderly may manifest itself differently from that seen in younger adults. Classic symptoms such as persistent sadness may be less pronounced, while other signs may predominate:

1. **Somatic symptoms**: Excessive fatigue, physical pain with no obvious organic cause, sleep disorders (insomnia or hypersomnia), significant weight loss or gain linked to changes in appetite.

2. **Anxiety and agitation**: Nervousness, irritability, impatience, psychomotor restlessness.

3. **Loss of interest and pleasure**: Markedly diminished interest in activities previously enjoyed, social withdrawal, apathy.

4. **Cognitive disorders**: Difficulty concentrating, memory problems, indecision, which may be mistaken for signs of dementia.

5. **Feelings of guilt and worthlessness**: feeling like a burden to loved ones, self-deprecation, recurring negative thoughts.

6. **Suicidal ideation**: morbid preoccupations, thoughts of death, verbal expressions of a wish not to live.

It's important to note that older people may minimize or not spontaneously express their emotional distress, making detection of depression more complex.

Risk factors for depression in the elderly

Several factors can contribute to the development of depression in the elderly:

1. **Stressful life events**: Bereavement of spouse or close friends, loss of independence, move to an institution, financial difficulties.

2. **Physical illnesses**: The presence of disabling chronic illnesses (e.g. cardiovascular disease, stroke, diabetes, cancer) can increase the risk of depression.

3. **Chronic pain**: Persistent pain can affect mood and quality of life.

4. **Social isolation**: lack of regular contact with family or friends, feelings of loneliness.

5. **Personal or family history of depression**: A genetic predisposition or history of mood disorders.

6. **Polymedication**: Certain medications can induce or aggravate depressive symptoms (e.g. certain antihypertensives, corticosteroids).

7. **Substance abuse**: Substance abuse can mask or exacerbate depression.

Consequences of depression in the elderly

Untreated depression can have serious repercussions:

1. **Functional decline**: Worsening dependency, reduced mobility, increased difficulty with activities of daily living.

2. **Aggravation of physical illness**: Depression can negatively influence the course of chronic illnesses,

reduce compliance with treatment and weaken the immune system.

3. **Increased suicidal risk**: Elderly people with depression have an increased risk of attempting suicide, often by more lethal means.

4. **Frequent hospitalizations**: Depression can lead to repeated hospitalizations, increasing the risk of nosocomial complications.

5. **Impaired quality of life**: mental distress, loss of hope, reduced general well-being.

Differential diagnosis

It is crucial to distinguish depression from other conditions that may present similar symptoms:

- **Dementias**: Depression-related cognitive disorders (depressive pseudodementia) can be reversible with appropriate treatment, unlike neurodegenerative dementias.

- **Secondary mood disorders**: Certain medical conditions (hypothyroidism, vitamin deficiencies) or medications can cause depressive symptoms.

The caregiver's role in detection and management

1. **Careful observation**: The caregiver is often the first to notice changes in the patient's behavior, mood or habits. They need to be alert to subtle signs of depression.

2. **Empathetic communication**: establishing a relationship of trust, encouraging patients to express their feelings, listening without judgment.

3. **Reporting to the care team**: Forward observations to nurses and doctors for further assessment.

4. **Support for daily activities**: Help patients maintain a routine, encouraging them to take part in pleasurable activities, even if they show little enthusiasm.

5. **Promoting autonomy**: Valuing patients' abilities, avoiding doing for them what they can do themselves, boosting their self-esteem.

6. **Preventing isolation**: Facilitate contact with family and friends, and organize social and group activities where possible.

7. **Monitoring therapeutic compliance**: help patients to follow their treatment, be vigilant for antidepressant side effects, which may be more pronounced in the elderly (e.g. orthostatic hypotension, confusion).

8. **Patient and family education**: Provide information on depression, destigmatize mental disorders, explain the importance of treatment.

Therapeutic interventions

1. **Pharmacological treatments**: Antidepressants can be effective, but require age-appropriate dosage and close monitoring for adverse effects. Response to treatment may be slower in the elderly.

2. **Psychotherapies**: Cognitive-behavioral therapies and interpersonal therapy can help modify negative thought patterns and improve interpersonal skills.

3. **Reminiscence therapies**: Encouraging the patient to recall positive memories can strengthen identity and emotional well-being.

4. **Physical activity**: Appropriate exercise improves mood, stimulates endorphin production and promotes sleep.

5. **Social interventions**: Participation in clubs, associations, volunteer activities to reinforce a sense of belonging and usefulness.

Prevention of mood disorders

1. **Promoting a healthy lifestyle**: balanced diet, regular physical activity, adequate sleep.

2. **Maintaining social ties**: Encouraging interaction, supporting family relationships and friendships.

3. **Involvement in meaningful activities**: Leisure, hobbies, cultural or spiritual activities that bring pleasure and meaning.

4. **Stress management**: relaxation techniques, meditation, deep breathing.

5. **Chronic disease monitoring**: Optimal management of physical ailments can reduce the risk of depression.

Special considerations

- **Stigma**: Mental disorders can be associated with stigmatization among the elderly. It's important to normalize the discussion around mental health.

- **Consent and autonomy**: Respect patients' decisions, even if they refuse treatment, while ensuring that they are well informed and understand the implications.

- **Cultural approach**: Take into account the beliefs, cultural values and religious practices that can influence the perception of depression and acceptance of treatment.

Impact on the caregiver

- **Emotional management**: Working with depressed patients can be stressful. It is important for caregivers to recognize their own emotions, and to seek support from colleagues or supervisors.

- **Ongoing training**: Regular training on mood disorders, communication strategies and support techniques.

- **Taking a step back**: Developing mechanisms to prevent burnout, such as sharing experiences and participating in support groups.

- Importance of social and family support

Social and family support plays a vital role in the lives of the elderly, influencing not only their emotional well-being, but also their physical and mental health. In the context of geriatrics, the caregiver must understand the importance of this support in order to offer holistic care adapted to the specific needs of elderly patients. Social isolation and loneliness are common problems among the elderly, and their impact on health is considerable. Social and family support can mitigate these adverse effects, promote autonomy and improve patients' quality of life.

The impact of social support on the health of the elderly

Regular social interaction and emotional support from family and friends help :

1. **Preventing depression and anxiety**: A strong social network provides a space for expressing feelings, sharing experiences and finding comfort, thus reducing the risk of mood disorders.

2. **Cognitive stimulation**: conversations, shared activities and social interaction stimulate cognitive functions, delaying cognitive decline and preventing dementia.

3. **Boosting the immune system**: Emotional well-being linked to social support has a positive effect on the immune system, increasing resistance to disease.

4. **Adopting healthy behaviors**: Family and friends can encourage a balanced diet, physical activity and compliance with medical treatments.

5. **Stress management**: Social support helps you cope with stressful situations, losses and changes associated with aging.

The family's role in supporting the elderly

The family is often the main source of support for the elderly. They can :

1. **Providing practical assistance**: Help with household chores, shopping, medical appointments, enabling patients to stay at home longer.

2. **Offer emotional support**: comforting presence, attentive listening, sharing memories and experiences.

3. **Participate in care decisions**: Collaborate with healthcare professionals to draw up an appropriate care plan that respects the patient's wishes.

4. **Monitoring health**: Detecting physical or mental changes, communicating with the care team when necessary.

5. **Encouraging autonomy**: supporting patients in activities they can carry out on their own, valuing their abilities, avoiding overprotection.

Family support challenges

However, the role of family caregiver can be a source of stress and fatigue:

- **Emotional and physical burden**: Caregivers can experience exhaustion, anxiety and depression, impacting on their own health.

- **Family conflicts**: Disagreements over care decisions and division of responsibilities can lead to tension.

- **Lack of knowledge**: Caregivers may feel helpless when faced with complex patient needs, requiring training or professional support.

The caregiver's role in social and family support

The caregiver can play a key role in reinforcing social and family support:

1. **Facilitating communication**: acting as an intermediary between patient, family and care team, ensuring clear transmission of information.

2. **Educate the family**: provide information on the disease, the care needed, support techniques, to strengthen the skills of caregivers.

3. **Support caregivers**: Listen to their concerns, direct them to support resources (self-help groups, respite services).

4. **Promote social activities**: Encourage patients to take part in community activities, clubs and associations, to broaden their social network.

5. **Adapting interventions**: Take into account the family and social context when planning care, respecting family dynamics and cultural preferences.

Strategies for strengthening social support

- **Creating links** : Encourage intergenerational encounters, volunteer visits and mentoring programs.

- **Use of technology**: Encourage the use of online communication (video calls, social networks) to maintain contact with distant relatives.

- **Group activities**: Organize workshops, outings and recreational activities in care facilities.

- **Community involvement**: Involve patients in local projects and adapted volunteer work, to reinforce their sense of usefulness and belonging.

Importance of culture and beliefs

Cultural values, traditions and religious beliefs influence the perception of social support:

- **Respecting cultural practices**: Adapting care to take account of specific customs, languages and rituals.

- **Integrating extended families**: In some cultures, the extended family plays a central role; involve all relevant members in care.

- **Celebrating events**: Organize celebrations and ceremonies that respect the patient's traditions, strengthening social ties.

Preventing social isolation

Social isolation has deleterious effects on the health of the elderly. The caregiver can :

- **Identify people at risk**: Identify patients without family support, living alone, with mobility difficulties.

- **Set up targeted interventions**: Home visits, teleassistance programs, partnerships with social services.

- **Encouraging participation**: Motivating patients to engage in activities adapted to their abilities and interests.

Professional, interdisciplinary support

- **Teamwork**: Collaborate with social workers, psychologists and animators to offer comprehensive support.

- **Continuing education**: Training in communication techniques, family conflict management and mediation.

- **Promoting supportive policies**: Advocate for resources and programs that support older people and their families.

Ethics and Deontology in Geriatrics

- Respect for dignity and autonomy

Respect for the dignity and autonomy of the elderly is a fundamental principle that guides all the actions of the geriatric caregiver. In a context where patients may be faced with a progressive loss of physical, cognitive or social capacities, it is essential to preserve their moral integrity and their sense of being considered as individuals in their own right. The caregiver plays a key role by adopting a person-centered approach, valuing their choices and promoting their self-determination.

Understanding dignity and autonomy

Dignity is a value intrinsic to every human being, regardless of age, health or social status. It implies respect, honor and recognition of the value of each individual. In geriatrics, dignity can be threatened by paternalistic attitudes, infantilization or a lack of consideration for patients' wishes and preferences.

Autonomy refers to a person's ability to make informed choices about his or her own life, including decisions about health and care. It encompasses the right to control one's body, one's environment and the interventions one receives. For older people, maintaining autonomy is crucial to preserving their identity, self-esteem and quality of life.

The caregiver's role in respecting dignity

1. **Respectful, empathetic communication**
   The caregiver must adopt a respectful approach to communication, using clear, appropriate and non-condescending language. Addressing the patient by name, addressing him or her as "sir" if so desired, and avoiding infantilizing nicknames are essential practices. Active listening enables us to understand the patient's needs, concerns and wishes, by offering a non-judgmental space for expression.

2. **Preserving privacy and confidentiality**
   During care, it is essential to respect the patient's physical and psychological privacy. This includes closing doors or drawing curtains during procedures, covering the patient as much as possible and warning him/her before any physical contact. The caregiver must

also ensure the confidentiality of personal information, avoiding any discussion of the patient's health in the presence of unauthorized third parties.

3. **Recognition of individuality**

    Each patient is a unique individual with his or her own history, values and preferences. The caregiver can personalize care by taking into account the patient's lifestyle, religious beliefs, cultural customs and interests. This approach reinforces the patient's sense of dignity and consideration.

Promoting autonomy

1. **Encouraging active participation**

    The caregiver must encourage the patient to take an active part in his/her care, according to his/her abilities. This may involve simple acts such as washing the face, dressing or feeding. Stimulating functional autonomy helps prevent a decline in physical abilities and boosts the patient's self-confidence.

2. **Respecting patients' choices and decisions**

    Patients have the right to make choices about their care and lifestyle. The caregiver must present the available options, explain the implications of each choice and respect the patient's decision, even if it differs from medical recommendations. This may include choice of clothing, daily activities or dietary preferences.

3. **Adapting the environment to promote autonomy**

    A safe, adapted environment enables patients to maintain their independence. The caregiver can help to adapt the living space by removing obstacles, installing technical aids such as grab bars, or adjusting the height of beds and chairs. Facilitating access to personal objects and means of communication also enhances the patient's independence.

Managing complex situations

1. **Informed consent and decision-making capacity**
   When the patient is capable of understanding information and making decisions, it is essential to provide clear explanations of the proposed care, and to obtain the patient's consent. In cases of cognitive impairment, the caregiver must adapt his or her communication, using visual aids or simple sentences, and check the patient's comprehension.

2. **Approach to refusing care**
   If the patient refuses care, the caregiver must try to understand the reasons for this refusal, which may be linked to pain, fear, fatigue or personal convictions. It is important to respect this choice, avoid confrontation and propose alternatives or postpone the treatment if possible. Collaboration with the multidisciplinary team is essential to adjust the care plan.

3. **Respect for advance directives and life project**
   If the patient has expressed advance wishes concerning the end of life, or specific directives concerning care, the caregiver must take these into account and ensure that the patient's wishes are respected. This shows respect for the patient's autonomy and freedom of decision.

Training and awareness-raising for caregivers

To guarantee respect for dignity and autonomy, the caregiver must:

- **Develop communication skills**: learn how to listen actively, manage difficult situations and adapt communication to the patient's abilities.
- **Legal and ethical aspects**: familiarize yourself with patients' rights, ethical charters and professional obligations.

- **Adopt a reflective attitude**: question your own practices, recognize prejudices or paternalistic attitudes, and engage in a continuous improvement process.
- **Collaborate with the multidisciplinary team**: share observations, participate in department meetings and contribute to the development of a patient-centered care plan.

Benefits of respecting dignity and autonomy

- **Improved quality of care**: A respected, autonomous patient is more likely to cooperate in care, communicate effectively and follow recommendations.
- **Enhanced psychological well-being**: Respect for dignity contributes to greater self-esteem, reduces anxiety and prevents mood disorders.
- **Preserving functional autonomy**: By encouraging independence, we maintain the patient's physical and cognitive capacities, thereby delaying dependency.
- **Trusting therapeutic relationship**: A respectful approach fosters a positive relationship between patient and caregiver, essential for effective care.

- Informed consent and patient rights

Informed consent and respect for patient rights are fundamental principles governing the therapeutic relationship between caregiver and patient. In geriatrics, where patients may present particular age-related vulnerabilities, it is essential for the caregiver to understand and respect these concepts to ensure ethical, legal and person-centered care.

Understanding informed consent

Informed consent is the process by which a fully informed and competent patient accepts or refuses a medical intervention. This consent is based on several key elements:

1. **Complete and comprehensible information**: Patients must receive all relevant information concerning their state of health, treatment options, potential risks and benefits, possible alternatives and the consequences of refusing care. Information must be presented in clear language, adapted to the patient's level of understanding.

2. **Ability to make decisions**: The patient must be able to understand the information provided, evaluate the options and make a free and voluntary decision. This implies that he/she is not under the influence of judgment-altering substances or undue pressure.

3. **Free and informed consent**: Consent must be given without coercion, manipulation or undue influence. Patients must feel that their choices are respected, whatever the context.

Role of the caregiver in the consent process

Although obtaining informed consent is generally the responsibility of the doctor or nurse, the caregiver plays an important role in this process:

- **Adapted communication**: As a professional in close contact with the patient, the caregiver can help clarify information, answer questions and check understanding. They can use visual aids, simple analogies or rephrase explanations to facilitate understanding.

- **Observation and reporting**: If the caregiver notices that the patient seems confused, anxious or unable to understand information, he/she should inform the care team for a reassessment of decision-making capacity.

- **Respecting patient decisions**: The caregiver must respect the patient's choice, whether to accept or refuse care, and avoid any form of judgment or pressure.

Special features in geriatrics

In the elderly, several factors can influence the consent process:

1. **Cognitive disorders**: The presence of dementia or cognitive disorders may affect the patient's ability to consent. In such cases, an assessment of decision-making capacity is necessary, and the use of a legal representative or trusted person may be considered.

2. **Sensory impairments**: Hearing or visual impairments can hamper communication. The caregiver must adapt his or her communication by speaking clearly, using hearing aids or large print.

3. **Cultural and linguistic barriers**: Cultural or linguistic differences can complicate understanding. It may be necessary to call on the services of an interpreter or cultural mediator.

4. **Increased vulnerability**: Elderly people may be more sensitive to outside influences, including family or institutional pressure. It is important to ensure that consent is truly free and informed.

Patient rights

Respect for patients' rights is enshrined in law and is an obligation for all healthcare professionals. The main rights include :

1. **Right to information**: Patients have the right to receive clear, fair and appropriate information about their state of health, proposed treatments and their progress.

2. **Right to privacy and confidentiality**: The patient's personal and medical information must be protected. The caregiver must take care not to divulge this information without the patient's consent.

3. **Right to consent to or refuse treatment** : Patients can accept or refuse any medical procedure. Refusal must be respected, even if it goes against medical recommendations.

4. **Right to pain relief**: Patients have the right to receive care aimed at relieving their pain and suffering.

5. **Right to appoint a trusted support person**: Patients can appoint a person to be consulted if their condition no longer allows them to express their wishes.

6. **Right of access to medical records**: Patients can consult their medical records and obtain a copy of the information contained therein.

7. **Right to dignity**: Patients must be treated with respect, without discrimination, and their dignity must be preserved in all circumstances.

Practical application for caregivers

1. **Promoting autonomy**: Encouraging patients to actively participate in their care, to ask questions and express their preferences.

2. **Open communication**: Establish a relationship of trust, listen to the patient without judgment, and facilitate dialogue with the healthcare team.

3. **Protecting confidentiality**: Ensure that patient discussions take place in appropriate locations and that files are secure.

4. **Vulnerability support**: Be alert to signs of abuse, coercion or undue influence, and act in accordance with institutional protocols to protect the patient.

5. **Continuing education**: Keep abreast of legal and ethical developments concerning patients' rights, and develop skills in clinical ethics.

Special situations

- **Temporary or permanent incapacity**: If the patient is incapable of giving consent (e.g. coma, acute confusion), necessary care can be provided in the patient's best interests, in compliance with advance directives or in consultation with the trusted support person.

- **Medical emergencies**: In emergency situations where consent cannot be obtained, care necessary to save the patient's life or preserve his or her health may be carried out without prior consent.

- **Refusal of care**: If a patient refuses essential care, the caregiver must respect this choice, while ensuring that the patient understands the consequences of his or her refusal. It is important to communicate this refusal to the nursing team, so that appropriate care can be taken.

Ethics and professional reflection

The caregiver may be faced with ethical dilemmas when it comes to respecting the patient's rights while ensuring their safety and well-being. In such situations, it is useful to :

- **Analyze the situation**: Identify ethical issues, conflicting values and professional obligations.

- **Consult the team**: Talk to colleagues, supervisors or ethics committees for perspective and advice.

- **Putting the patient first**: Keep in mind that respecting the patient's wishes and rights is paramount, while taking care to do no harm.

- Confidentiality and professional secrecy

Confidentiality and professional secrecy are essential pillars of nursing practice, particularly in geriatrics, where elderly patients are often vulnerable and dependent on the respect and trust of healthcare professionals. For the caregiver, these concepts are of major importance, as they guarantee respect for patient privacy, protect personal information and reinforce the relationship of trust essential to quality care.

Understanding confidentiality and professional secrecy

Confidentiality refers to the obligation not to divulge personal and medical information about a patient to unauthorized third parties. It encompasses all data obtained within the therapeutic relationship, whether medical, psychological or social in nature.

Professional secrecy is a legal and ethical obligation that requires healthcare professionals to keep secret information entrusted to them by patients or discovered in the course of their duties. In France, this obligation is enshrined in the Public Health Code, and any breach is punishable by law.

The importance of professional secrecy in geriatrics

Elderly patients may present special situations that make confidentiality even more crucial:

- **Increased vulnerability**: Elderly people may be more dependent, physically and psychologically fragile, and therefore more likely to be affected by a violation of their privacy.
- **Complexity of family situations**: Family dynamics can be complex, with potential conflicts or diverging interests between family members.
- **Protection against abuse**: Respect for professional secrecy helps protect patients against abuse, discrimination or stigmatization.

The caregiver's role in respecting confidentiality

1. **Managing personal information**
   The caregiver is often at the forefront of gathering sensitive information during daily care. They must :

   - **Collect only the information needed** to manage the patient.
   - **Ensure data security**: Don't leave documents containing personal information lying around, lock computer files, respect document storage and destruction protocols.

2. **Communication with the care team**

   - **Relevant sharing**: Transmit to colleagues only the information required for continuity of care.
   - **Discretion**: Avoid discussing patients in public places or within earshot of unauthorized persons (corridors, elevators, canteens).

3. **Interaction with families and friends**
    - **Respecting the patient's wishes**: Only share information with the family with the patient's explicit consent.
    - **Handling requests for information**: If a family member requests information, the caregiver must check the patient's authorization or refer the person to a line manager or the doctor in charge.

4. **Use of new technologies**
    - **Caution with electronic devices**: Do not record or distribute photos, videos or patient information via cell phones or social networks.
    - **Data protection**: Use secure passwords, log out of computer sessions after use.

Exceptional situations and waiver of professional secrecy

Professional secrecy is a general obligation, but certain situations may require a legal exemption:

- **Danger to the patient or others**: If the patient presents an imminent risk to him/herself or others (e.g. suicidal thoughts, violence), the caregiver must alert the competent authorities or the medical team.
- **Reporting abuse**: If abuse of an elderly person is suspected or observed, the caregiver has a duty to report the facts to the authorities, in accordance with established procedures.
- **Judicial requisitions**: If the courts request information as part of an investigation, the professional must respond within the legal limits.

In such cases, it is essential to follow institutional protocols and refer to line management or legal services to act appropriately.

Consequences of breaching professional secrecy

Breach of professional secrecy may result in :

- **Penalties**: In France, the disclosure of information covered by professional secrecy is punishable by law (article 226-13 of the Penal Code) by up to one year's imprisonment and a 15,000 euro fine.
- **Disciplinary measures**: Employers may take disciplinary action against caregivers, up to and including dismissal.
- **Damage to the relationship of trust**: Such a violation can break the trust between patient and caregiver, harming the quality of care and the image of the facility.

Strategies for maintaining confidentiality on a daily basis

1. **Training and awareness-raising**

    - **Know your legal and ethical obligations**: Keep abreast of legal texts, professional charters and internal regulations.
    - **Participate in ongoing training** on confidentiality, data management and professional ethics.

2. **Adopting exemplary behavior**

    - **Setting an example**: By adopting a discreet, professional attitude, caregivers encourage their colleagues to do the same.
    - **Responding to breaches**: If a colleague discloses inappropriate information, the caregiver must respectfully call him or her to order or inform a superior.

3. **Appropriate use of workspaces**

    o **Preserve privacy during care**: Close doors, use screens, keep voices low.
    o **Avoid inappropriate conversations** in public places or in the presence of other patients.

4. **Document and media management**

    o **Put files away** after consultation, do not leave them accessible to unauthorized persons.
    o **Destroy documents** containing sensitive information according to established procedures (shredders, secure containers).

5. **Patient communication**

    o **Inform patients** of their confidentiality rights.
    o **Obtain consent** before sharing information with third parties, including family if necessary.

The caregiver's role in the multidisciplinary team

- **Respectful collaboration**: Share relevant information with the care team in a confidential manner.
- **Mutual support**: Supporting each other to ensure professional secrecy, sharing best practices.

Chapter 2

The role of the caregiver in geriatrics

Skills and Qualifications

- Basic medical knowledge

To work effectively as a geriatric caregiver, it is essential to have a sound basic medical knowledge. This knowledge enables you to understand the mechanisms of the human body, recognize important clinical signs and work closely with the nursing team. It is the foundation on which the practical and interpersonal skills needed to care for the elderly are built.

1. Human anatomy and physiology

An understanding of anatomy and physiology is fundamental to understanding the normal functioning of the human body and identifying abnormalities. Here are the main systems you need to know about:

- **Cardiovascular system**: Understanding the structure of the heart, blood vessels and blood circulation enables us to grasp the mechanisms of hypertension, heart failure and coronary heart disease.

- **Respiratory system**: Knowing the anatomy of the airways, the lungs and the gas exchange process is crucial to recognizing the signs of respiratory distress, chronic obstructive pulmonary disease (COPD) and lung infections.

- **Nervous system**: Understanding the functioning of the central and peripheral nervous system helps to understand neurological disorders, stroke and neurodegenerative diseases such as Alzheimer's and Parkinson's.

- **Musculoskeletal system**: Knowledge of bones, muscles and joints is essential for preventing falls, managing arthritic pain and promoting mobility.

- **Digestive system**: Understanding the process of digestion and nutrient absorption helps to monitor nutritional status, prevent constipation and recognize signs of gastrointestinal disorders.

- **Urinary system**: Understanding kidney function and the process of urine formation is important for monitoring hydration, preventing urinary tract infections and detecting signs of kidney failure.

- **Endocrine system**: Understanding the role of hormones helps to understand diseases such as diabetes, hypothyroidism and age-related hormonal imbalances.

- **Immune system**: Understanding the body's defense mechanisms is key to understanding the importance of vaccinations, infection prevention and inflammatory reactions.

2. Vital signs and clinical parameters

Controlling vital signs is essential for assessing the patient's state of health and rapidly detecting any abnormalities:

- **Body temperature**: Understand normal variations and the implications of fever or hypothermia.

- **Heart rate**: Know how to measure pulse, recognize normal rhythms and anomalies such as tachycardia or bradycardia.

- **Respiratory rate**: Assess breathing, identify dyspnea, apnea or hyperventilation.

- **Blood pressure**: Measure blood pressure, understand normal values and identify hypertension or hypotension.

- **Oxygen saturation**: Use a saturometer to check blood oxygenation and identify hypoxia.

3. Common pathologies in the elderly

Knowing the most common diseases allows you to monitor symptoms, prevent complications and support the patient:

- **Cardiovascular diseases**: high blood pressure, heart failure, coronary heart disease, stroke.

- **Metabolic disorders**: type 2 diabetes, dyslipidemia, obesity.

- **Respiratory diseases**: COPD, asthma, pulmonary infections.

- **Neurological disorders**: dementia, Parkinson's disease, epilepsy.

- **Musculoskeletal disorders**: osteoarthritis, osteoporosis, fractures.

- **Sensory disorders**: reduced vision (cataracts, macular degeneration), hearing loss.

- **Kidney diseases**: chronic renal failure, urinary tract infections.

- **Gastrointestinal disorders**: Constipation, ulcers, liver disease.

- **Mental disorders**: depression, anxiety, sleep disorders.

4. Pharmacological principles

A basic understanding of pharmacology is needed to help with medication management, while respecting the role of the nurse:

- **Drug classes** : Know the main types of drugs used in geriatrics (antihypertensives, antidiabetics, analgesics, anticoagulants, psychotropics).

- **Routes of administration**: Understand the different routes (oral, cutaneous, parenteral) and associated precautions.

- **Side effects**: Watch out for signs of common side effects, such as drowsiness, dizziness and digestive disorders.

- **Drug interactions**: Be aware that polymedication can lead to interactions, requiring closer monitoring.

- **Therapeutic compliance**: Encourage patients to follow their treatment, explain the importance of regularity and report any refusals or omissions.

5. Hygiene and infection control

Hygiene principles are fundamental to preventing the spread of infections, especially in elderly people with weakened immune systems:

- **Hand hygiene**: mastering hand-washing techniques, using hydroalcoholic solutions.

- **Use of personal protective equipment**: gloves, masks, gowns according to protocols.

- **Standard precautions**: Apply basic measures for all patients, regardless of diagnosis.

- **Waste management**: Proper disposal of infectious waste, sharps.

- **Disinfection of surfaces and equipment**: Regular cleaning of care areas to reduce risks.

6. Nutrition and hydration

Nutritional status is a major determinant of health in the elderly:

- **Specific nutritional needs**: Understand that protein, vitamin and mineral requirements may change with age.

- **Signs of undernutrition**: involuntary weight loss, muscle weakness, apathy.

- **Hydration**: Recognize signs of dehydration (dry mouth, hypotension, confusion) and encourage adequate fluid intake.

- **Diet adaptation**: consistency of food to prevent false routes, compliance with special diets (diabetic, low-calorie).

7. Basic care and patient comfort

Ensuring the patient's comfort and well-being is an essential component of care:

- **Mobilization and pressure sore prevention**: Techniques for changing positions, use of adapted mattresses, preventive massages.

- **Personal grooming and hygiene**: help with grooming in a dignified manner, skin care, oral hygiene.

- **Dressing and undressing**: Appropriate assistance, choice of comfortable, safe clothing.

- **Urinary and faecal elimination**: Assistance with toilet use, elimination monitoring, incontinence prevention.

- **Pain management**: Recognize the signs of pain, assess its intensity and inform the care team.

8. First aid

In the event of an emergency, the caregiver must know how to react quickly while awaiting medical intervention:

- **Recognize emergency situations**: fainting, falls, cardiac arrest, choking.

- **First aid techniques**: Lateral position, basic cardiopulmonary resuscitation, airway clearance.

- **Calling for help**: Know who to contact, provide clear, precise information.

9. Therapeutic communication

Communication is a powerful therapeutic tool:

- **Active listening**: Pay attention, show empathy, encourage the patient to express him/herself.

- **Language adaptation**: using simple words, ensuring comprehension, taking into account cognitive or sensory impairments.

- **Non-verbal**: Pay attention to gestures, facial expressions and the patient's posture.

- **Respect and benevolence**: Creating a climate of trust, respecting patients' choices and dignity.

10. Multidisciplinary teamwork

The caregiver is an integral part of the care team:

- **Written and verbal communications**: Effectively communicate observations, status changes and incidents.

- **Collaboration**: working in synergy with nurses, doctors, physiotherapists and dieticians.

- **Knowledge of roles and limits**: Respect each other's skills, don't overstep your boundaries.

- Relational and communication skills

Relational and communication skills are central to the profession of geriatric caregiver. Indeed, the quality of the relationship established between the caregiver and the elderly patient directly influences the well-being, safety and effectiveness of the care provided. In a context where the elderly may face physical, cognitive or emotional difficulties, appropriate and empathetic communication is essential to meet their specific needs and preserve their dignity.

The importance of communication in geriatrics

Communicating with the elderly has its own particularities, due to the physiological and psychological changes associated with aging. Sensory problems, such as reduced hearing or vision, cognitive disorders, such as dementia, or emotional barriers due to isolation or depression, can hamper exchanges. The caregiver must therefore develop specific skills to establish a relationship of trust and facilitate mutual understanding.

Verbal communication skills

1. **Clarity and simplicity of language**: Use accessible vocabulary, short sentences and avoid medical jargon. This helps patients understand the information conveyed and feel included in the care process.

2. **Adapting tone and rhythm**: Speak clearly, at an appropriate volume, articulating well, especially in the presence of hearing difficulties. Adapt the pace of

speech to give the patient time to process the information.

3. **Use of open-ended questions**: Encourage patients to express themselves freely by asking questions that require more than a yes or no answer. This encourages the expression of needs, concerns and feelings.

4. **Reformulation and validation**: Reformulate the patient's words to ensure mutual understanding and show that they are being taken into account.

Non-verbal communication skills

1. **Eye contact**: Maintain a kind, attentive gaze to establish a connection and show interest. This is particularly important for hearing-impaired patients who can rely on lip-reading.

2. **Facial expressions and gestures**: Adopt warm facial expressions and open, welcoming gestures. Smiles, nods and signs of approval reinforce the verbal message.

3. **Proxemia**: Respect the patient's personal distance, yet be close enough to communicate effectively. Adapt your position, for example by sitting at the same height as the bed-ridden patient.

4. **Therapeutic touch**: Using physical contact in appropriate ways to bring comfort, such as placing a hand on the shoulder, while respecting the patient's limits.

Active listening and empathy

Active listening is an essential skill that involves total attention to the patient's words, without interruption or judgment. It manifests itself in :

- **Focus on the patient's speech**: Put aside your own thoughts and focus on what the patient is saying.

- **Verbal and non-verbal responses**: Use signs to show that you're following the thread of the conversation, such as nodding or using appropriate interjections.

- **Empathy**: Putting yourself in the patient's shoes to understand their emotions and perspectives. Empathy enables us to respond appropriately to the patient's emotional needs.

Managing difficult situations

The caregiver may be confronted with complex situations, such as aggressiveness, anxiety or confusion on the part of the patient. To deal with them :

- **Remain calm and patient**: Don't react impulsively, keep a serene attitude to calm the situation.

- **Identify the causes**: Seek to understand the underlying reasons for the behavior, whether it's pain, fear or frustration.

- **Use detour techniques**: steer the conversation towards soothing or positive topics to divert the patient's attention.

- **Involve the team**: Don't hesitate to ask colleagues or superiors for support when needed.

Communication with cognitively impaired patients

People with dementia or other cognitive disorders require a special approach:

- **Simplify language**: Use simple sentences, one idea at a time, and avoid complex questions.

- **Reduce distractions**: Communicate in a calm environment to minimize disruptive stimuli.

- **Repeat and rephrase**: Don't hesitate to repeat information consistently, keeping your tone neutral.

- **Use visual aids**: Use images, objects or gestures to facilitate understanding.

Working with family and friends

Communication is not limited to the patient, but also includes families:

- **Inform tactfully**: Pass on relevant information about the patient's condition, while respecting confidentiality and patient consent.

- **Listen to concerns**: Welcome the questions and feelings of loved ones, who may be anxious or worried.

- **Involving caregivers**: Encourage the participation of relatives in care, according to the patient's wishes, to reinforce social support.

Communication within the care team

Good inter-professional communication is essential:

- **Clear, precise communication**: Share important patient information in a structured manner, both orally and in writing.

- **Respect and collaboration**: Foster a climate of trust between colleagues, by valuing each person's skills.

- **Conflict management**: deal with disagreements constructively, emphasizing dialogue and the search for solutions.

Continuing education and skills development

Relational and communication skills can be improved by :

- **Self-evaluation**: Reflect on your practice, identify strengths and areas for improvement.

- **Specific training**: Participate in workshops or training courses on communication, active listening and emotion management.

- **Supervision and feedback**: Solicit feedback from colleagues and superiors to help you progress.

- Stress management and resilience

Managing stress and developing resilience are essential skills for geriatric caregivers, given the emotional and physical challenges inherent in their profession. On a daily basis, caregivers are confronted with complex situations, such as caring for patients with chronic illnesses, managing pain, providing end-of-life support, and interacting with grieving families. These responsibilities can generate high levels of stress, which can affect their personal well-being and professional effectiveness. It is therefore essential to adopt stress management strategies and cultivate resilience to maintain a healthy and sustainable practice.

Understanding stress in the geriatric context

Stress is the body's natural reaction to situations perceived as demanding or threatening. In the context of geriatric work, stress can arise from a variety of sources: work overload, time pressure, emotional constraints linked to patient suffering, complexity of care, and sometimes lack of recognition. In addition, caregivers may experience moral stress when faced with ethical dilemmas or end-of-life situations.

The manifestations of stress can be physical (fatigue, sleep disorders, muscular tension), emotional (anxiety, irritability, sadness) or behavioral (disengagement, professional errors). In the long term, poorly managed stress can lead to burn-out, characterized by emotional fatigue, depersonalization and a diminished sense of accomplishment.

Stress management strategies

To prevent and manage stress, caregivers can implement several effective strategies:

1. **Self-assessment and awareness**
   It's important to recognize the signs of stress and identify specific sources. Regular self-assessment enables you to become aware of your emotional and physical state, making it easier to take appropriate action.

2. **Relaxation techniques**
   Methods such as deep breathing, meditation, progressive muscle relaxation or yoga can help reduce tension and promote a state of calm. These techniques can be practiced daily, even for short periods.

3. **Time management and organization**
   Effective task planning helps reduce work overload and the feeling of being overwhelmed. Prioritizing activities, delegating where possible and establishing a work-life balance are key.

4. **Social and professional support**
   Sharing with trusted colleagues, supervisors or friends allows you to express frustrations, receive advice and feel supported. Participating in discussion or

supervision groups can also provide a space for exchanging experiences and strategies.

5. **Ongoing training**
   Acquiring new skills and keeping abreast of best practices boosts self-confidence and professional effectiveness, reducing the stress associated with uncertainty or perceived incompetence.

6. **Taking personal responsibility**
   Maintaining a healthy lifestyle is essential: a balanced diet, sufficient sleep and regular exercise all contribute to better resistance to stress.

7. **Limiting modifiable stress factors**
   Identify aspects of work that can be changed and work with the team or management to improve conditions, such as task allocation, scheduling, or access to necessary resources.

Building resilience

Resilience is the ability to adapt positively in the face of adversity, to bounce back from difficult situations and maintain an optimal level of functioning. For caregivers, developing resilience not only enables them to manage stress, but also to find meaning and satisfaction in their work despite the challenges.

Factors promoting resilience

1. **Positive attitude and optimism**
   Cultivating a positive outlook, seeking out the satisfying aspects of work, celebrating small victories and appreciating moments of gratitude can boost motivation and well-being.

2. **Sense of purpose and meaning**
   Remembering the deeper reasons for choosing this

profession, recognizing the positive impact on patients and their families, and aligning daily actions with personal values all contribute to a sense of fulfillment.

3. **Flexibility and adaptation**
   Developing the ability to adapt to change, accept unexpected situations and modify plans accordingly helps reduce frustration and stress.

4. **Problem-solving skills**
   Tackling challenges proactively, seeking creative solutions and learning from each experience builds confidence in one's abilities.

5. **Strong support network**
   Positive relationships with colleagues, friends and family provide emotional and practical support in times of need.

6. **Self-compassion**
   Being kind to yourself, recognizing your limits, accepting mistakes as learning opportunities and avoiding excessive self-criticism all contribute to better mental health.

Integrating stress management and resilience into professional practice

Healthcare facilities can also play a role in supporting caregivers in these areas:

- **Workplace wellness programs**
  Set up initiatives to promote mental health, such as stress management workshops, relaxation sessions or group physical activities.

- **Encouraging open communication**
  Foster an environment where caregivers feel

comfortable expressing their concerns, without fear of judgment or negative repercussions.

- **Recognition and appreciation**
Acknowledging work accomplished, offering positive feedback and valuing individual and collective contributions boost morale and commitment.

- **Access to professional resources**
Provide psychological support, such as access to counselors or psychologists, and information on resources available to help in case of difficulties.

Responsibilities and role limits

- Authorized activities and delegated acts

The profession of caregiver is governed by a legal and regulatory framework that precisely defines the authorized activities and acts that can be delegated by the nurse or doctor. Understanding these limits is essential if you are to work safely, provide quality care and meet your professional obligations. In the context of geriatrics, where the needs of elderly patients are complex and varied, the caregiver plays a crucial role in close collaboration with the nursing team.

Legal and regulatory framework

In France, the role of the caregiver is defined by the Public Health Code and related regulations. Caregivers work under the responsibility of the nurse, in accordance with article R.4311-4 of the Public Health Code, which specifies the acts they are authorized to perform.

Authorized caregiver activities

Caregivers contribute to the hygiene, comfort and well-being of patients. Their main activities include :

1. **Hygiene and comfort care**: Help with washing, mouth care, dressing and undressing, while respecting the patient's privacy and dignity.

2. **Help with feeding and hydration**: Accompany patients during meals, take care of their nutritional needs, comply with prescribed diets and prevent the risk of false feeds.

3. **Mobilization and positioning**: Help patients move around and change position to prevent pressure sores, use appropriate technical aids and ensure their safety.

4. **Clinical status monitoring**: Observe clinical signs (temperature, pulse, respiration), detect changes in the patient's state of health and inform the nurse.

5. **Environmental maintenance**: Ensuring the cleanliness of the patient's living space, managing linen, ensuring the comfort and safety of the premises.

6. **Relational support**: Listening to patients, comforting them, encouraging exchanges, helping to maintain their morale and psychological well-being.

7. **Welcome and integration**: Facilitate the patient's arrival on the ward, inform him/her about how the establishment works, introduce the care team.

8. **Transmitting information**: communicating accurately and completely with the care team, taking part in written and oral communications, respecting professional secrecy.

Acts delegated by the nurse

Nurses may delegate certain actions to caregivers, in compliance with regulations and under their own responsibility. These delegated acts must meet several conditions:

- **Competence of the caregiver** : The caregiver must be adequately trained and able to perform the procedure safely.

- **No contraindications**: The patient must be in a stable condition, with no particular risk associated with the delegated procedure.

- **Monitoring and evaluation**: The nurse must ensure that the procedure is carried out correctly, and be available to intervene if necessary.

Among the acts that can be delegated are :

1. **Measurement of vital parameters**: Temperature, pulse, blood pressure, respiratory rate, under the nurse's supervision.

2. **Medication assistance**: Distribution of non-injectable medications prepared by the nurse, ensuring compliance and monitoring adverse effects.

3. **Elimination care**: Placement of bedpans, assistance with toilet use, diuresis and stool monitoring, management of elimination devices (urine bags, stomas) after specific training.

4. **Pressure sore prevention**: Preventive massages, application of protective creams, use of suitable supports.

5. **Specialized nursing care**: Participation in the care of patients with cognitive disorders, under the guidance of the nurse and after appropriate training.

Limits of delegated acts

It is important to note that certain procedures are strictly reserved for nurses or doctors, and can under no circumstances be delegated to a caregiver. These procedures include

- **Administration of injectable drugs**: Subcutaneous, intramuscular or intravenous injections are the exclusive responsibility of the nurse.

- **Infusion placement**: Placement of peripheral or central venous catheters.

- **Blood sampling**: Blood sampling requires specific training and legal authorization.

- **Specialized technical care**: Complex dressings, bladder catheterization, tracheal aspirations.

- **Nursing diagnosis**: Assessing needs, planning care and making clinical decisions are all part of the nurse's job.

Responsibilities and interprofessional collaboration

The caregiver works under the responsibility of the nurse, which implies close collaboration and effective communication. They must respect established protocols, medical prescriptions and the nurse's directives. In case of doubt or unusual situation, it is essential to consult the nurse before acting.

The caregiver is also liable for professional negligence. They must exercise diligence, competence and caution, in accordance with the rules of the art and good practice.

Continuing education and skills development

To ensure quality care and broaden their skills, caregivers are encouraged to take part in ongoing training courses. This training may cover :

- **New care techniques**: Update your knowledge of protocols, medical devices and therapeutic approaches.

- **Specific care**: Training in pain management, palliative care and communication with dementia patients.

- **Hygiene and infection prevention**: Reinforcing hand hygiene, asepsis and epidemic management practices.

- **Care safety**: fall prevention, risk management, use of personal protective equipment.

Ethics and respect for the patient

In all their activities, caregivers must act with respect, kindness and in accordance with the ethical principles of the profession. They must take care to :

- **Respect the patient's dignity**: Preserve privacy, respect patient choices and values.

- **Ensuring confidentiality**: Protecting personal and medical information, respecting professional secrecy.

- **Promoting autonomy**: Encouraging patients to participate in their own care and maintain their functional abilities.

- Collaboration with the care team

Collaboration with the nursing team is fundamental to the practice of the geriatric caregiver. It is the foundation on which the quality of care provided to the elderly rests, promoting comprehensive, coherent, patient-centered care. In a context where patients' needs are complex and multi-dimensional, synergy between different healthcare professionals is essential to ensure an appropriate and effective response.

The importance of interprofessional collaboration

The elderly often present multiple pathologies, as well as physical, cognitive and social frailties, requiring a multidisciplinary approach. Collaboration within the care team makes it possible to :

1. **Ensuring continuity of care**: By sharing relevant information, each team member can adapt his or her interventions to the patient's evolving condition, avoiding redundancies or omissions.

2. **Optimizing the quality of care**: pooling the skills and perspectives of each professional enriches care, enabling innovative, customized solutions to be proposed.

3. **Preventing errors and incidents**: Effective communication reduces the risk of medication errors, poor follow-up and avoidable complications.

4. **Promoting patient well-being**: By working together, the team creates a reassuring environment for patients, who feel supported and understood as a whole.

The caregiver's role in the care team

The caregiver occupies a central position in the team, thanks to his or her proximity to the patient and intimate knowledge of his or her daily needs. Collaborative responsibilities include :

1. **Information transmission**

    ◦ **Clinical observations**: The caregiver is often the first to detect changes in the patient's condition, such as signs of pain, confusion, fatigue or distress. It is essential that he/she communicates these observations to the nurse or physician for further assessment.

    ◦ **Written and oral communications**: Taking an active part in communications during shift changeovers, by providing precise, objective and relevant information, helps to ensure continuity of care between teams.

2. **Participation in department meetings**

    ◦ **Interdisciplinary exchanges**: department meetings and wrap-up sessions are opportunities for caregivers to share their observations, put forward ideas and contribute to the development of the care plan.

    ◦ **Sharing experiences**: Discussing complex cases, sharing successes and difficulties encountered, encourages collective learning and improved practices.

3. **Coordination of interventions**

    ◦ **Care planning**: Collaborate with nurses, physiotherapists, occupational therapists and other professionals to organize care effectively, taking into account each person's priorities and constraints.

    ◦ **Adapting to the patient's needs**: Based on feedback from the team, adjust interventions to better meet the patient's expectations, for example by modifying care schedules to respect his or her rhythm of life.

4. **Support for colleagues**

    - **Working in pairs**: For difficult mobilizations or high-risk situations, the caregiver can call on the help of a colleague to ensure the safety of both patient and caregiver.

    - **Sharing knowledge**: passing on specific skills, particularly in communicating with cognitively impaired patients, helps to strengthen the team's capabilities.

Effective team communication

Clear, respectful communication is the key to successful collaboration. To achieve this, the caregiver must:

1. **Adopting a professional attitude**

    - **Mutual respect**: Treat each team member with consideration, recognize each other's skills and avoid judgment or non-constructive criticism.

    - **Open-mindedness**: Be receptive to suggestions, accept feedback and criticism in a positive way to improve your practice.

2. **Use appropriate communication tools**

    - **Care records**: Record important information clearly, concisely and in accordance with established protocols.

    - **Digital media**: Master care management software and internal communication applications, while respecting data confidentiality and security rules.

3. **Managing conflict constructively**

    - **Seeking solutions**: In the event of disagreement, encourage dialogue, express points of view assertively and seek a compromise in the patient's best interests.

    - **Mediation**: If necessary, call on a neutral third party, such as a line manager, to help resolve the conflict.

Collaboration with other healthcare professionals

In addition to the nursing team, the caregiver interacts with various professionals:

1. **Doctors**

    - **Relevant information**: Transmit to physicians significant clinical observations that may influence diagnosis or treatment.

    - **Prescription follow-up**: Ensure the implementation of medical prescriptions, in collaboration with the nurse.

2. **Physiotherapists and occupational therapists**

    - **Rehabilitation support**: Helping the patient with exercises, encouraging participation, following instructions to promote functional recovery.

    - **Adapting the environment**: Working together to adapt the patient's home or bedroom, installing technical aids to facilitate daily activities.

3. **Psychologists**

    - **Behavioral observation**: Report mood swings, signs of anxiety or depression that may require psychological intervention.
    - **Emotional support**: Apply the psychologist's recommendations to improve the patient's mental well-being.

4. **Social workers**

    - **Resource referral**: Inform the social worker of the patient's needs in terms of financial assistance, home services or accommodation.
    - **Coordinating procedures**: Facilitating communication between patients, their families and social services.

Continuing education and professional development

Effective collaboration also relies on skills development:

1. **Participation in training courses**

    - **Knowledge updates**: Keep abreast of changes in care practices, protocols and regulations.
    - **Interprofessional workshops**: Participate in joint training sessions with other professionals to strengthen team cohesion.

2. **Supervision and tutoring**

    ○ **Supporting new arrivals**: Welcoming trainees or new colleagues, sharing best practices, fostering their integration.

    ○ **Reflecting on practice**: Engaging in discussions on complex cases, analyzing situations to improve future interventions.

Positive impact on quality of care

Harmonious collaboration within the care team means :

1. **Improved patient satisfaction**

    ○ **Personalized care**: By coordinating efforts, the team can offer care tailored to the patient's specific needs, enhancing comfort and confidence.

    ○ **Reactivity**: Fluid communication enables rapid response to changes in the patient's condition, preventing complications.

2. **Organizational efficiency**

    ○ **Optimization of resources**: by distributing tasks fairly, the team avoids overloading and improves the efficiency of interventions.

    ○ **Reducing errors**: Mutual monitoring and information sharing reduce the risk of medication errors or negligence.

3. **Positive work climate**

    ○ **Motivation and commitment**: A close-knit team fosters a pleasant working environment, encouraging everyone to get involved.

    ○ **Professional development**: Collaboration offers opportunities for mutual learning and skill progression.

- Legal and professional liability

Legal and professional responsibility is a fundamental pillar of the practice of geriatric caregivers. It encompasses all the legal, ethical and deontological obligations that guide the actions of these healthcare professionals. Understanding and respecting these responsibilities is essential to ensuring quality care, protecting patients' rights and guaranteeing the legal security of caregivers themselves. In a context where the elderly are often vulnerable, it is crucial that caregivers exercise their profession with rigor, integrity and conscientiousness.

Legal framework for the caregiver profession

In France, the profession of caregiver is regulated by the Public Health Code, which defines the competencies, authorized acts and professional obligations of caregivers. Caregivers work under the responsibility of nurses, in accordance with article R.4311-4 of the Public Health Code. This legal framework specifies the limits of their field of action and the conditions under which they can work with patients.

Furthermore, caregivers are subject to the same legal obligations as all healthcare professionals, notably in terms of professional secrecy, respect for patient rights, and civil and criminal liability.

Civil liability

The caregiver's civil liability concerns damage caused to a patient as a result of fault, negligence or imprudence in the performance of his or her duties. If a patient suffers harm as a result of an act or omission by the caregiver, the latter may be liable to pay compensation.

For example, if a caregiver causes a patient to fall by failing to follow mobilization protocols, he or she may be held liable for the injuries caused. The aim of civil liability is to compensate the victim for the damage suffered, generally in the form of financial compensation.

Criminal liability

Criminal liability involves penalties for offenses defined by law, such as breach of professional secrecy, abuse, manslaughter or deliberately endangering the life of others. Caregivers may be subject to criminal prosecution if they commit acts contrary to the law in the course of their professional activity.

For example, disclosing confidential information about a patient is a criminal offence punishable under Article 226-13 of the French Penal Code. Similarly, physical or psychological mistreatment of a vulnerable person is severely punished.

Professional and ethical obligations

In addition to their legal obligations, caregivers are bound by ethical and deontological principles that guide their practice:

1. **Respecting patients' dignity and rights**
   Caregivers must treat every patient with respect, without discrimination, preserving their dignity, privacy and autonomy. They must respect patients' choices, including their right to consent to or refuse care.

2. **Professional secrecy**
   Professional secrecy is a fundamental obligation. It prohibits the disclosure of any personal information concerning the patient, obtained in the course of professional practice. This obligation is designed to protect the patient's privacy and establish a relationship of trust.

3. **Competence and up-to-date knowledge**
   Caregivers have a duty to perform their duties competently and diligently. They must keep their knowledge and skills up to date, in particular by taking part in ongoing training, to ensure quality care in line with evolving practices.

4. **Duty of care and safety**
   They must take all necessary precautions to ensure patient safety, by complying with protocols, hygiene procedures and rules of good practice. This includes preventing infections, managing care-related risks and carefully monitoring patients' condition.

5. **Interprofessional collaboration**
   Caregivers must work closely with the nursing team, respecting each other's skills and responsibilities. They must communicate effectively and professionally, sharing information relevant to patient care.

Special situations and obligations

1. **Reporting situations of abuse**
   Caregivers have a legal obligation to report situations of abuse or endangerment involving vulnerable patients. This may include neglect, physical, psychological or financial abuse. Reporting must be made to the appropriate authorities, following established procedures.

2. **Managing refusal of care**
    If a patient refuses care, the caregiver must respect his or her decision, after ensuring that the patient has been fully informed of the consequences. He/she must inform the nurse or doctor in charge to assess the situation and determine the action to be taken.

3. **Prohibition of the illegal practice of medicine or nursing**
    The caregiver must ensure that he/she does not perform acts reserved for doctors or nurses, such as diagnostic procedures, prescribing treatments, administering injectable medicines or performing specific unauthorized technical care.

Consequences of non-compliance

Failure to comply with legal and professional obligations can have serious consequences for the caregiver:

- **Disciplinary sanctions**: Employers can take disciplinary measures ranging from a warning to dismissal for serious misconduct.
- **Criminal sanctions**: In the event of a breach of the law, the caregiver may be fined, imprisoned or disqualified.
- **Civil liability**: He may be required to pay compensation for damage caused to the patient.
- **Damage to professional reputation**: Breaches can affect the credibility and trust placed in the caregiver by patients, colleagues and employers.

Preventing and managing legal risks

To protect themselves and work safely, caregivers must :

1. **Know the legal framework**
   Familiarize yourself with the laws, regulations and professional texts governing your practice. This includes the French Public Health Code, the Code of Ethics for Nurses (which also guides caregivers), and the facility's internal protocols.

2. **Respect procedures and protocols**
   Rigorously apply care procedures, hygiene rules, safety protocols and the directives of the care team. This reduces the risk of errors and malpractice.

3. **Document actions**
   Accurately and objectively record the care provided, clinical observations and any incidents in care records. Good traceability is essential to ensure continuity of care and protection in the event of litigation.

4. **Communicating effectively**
   Maintain clear, professional communication with the nursing team, patients and families. In case of doubt or complex situations, it is important to consult the nurse or doctor.

5. **Participate in ongoing training**
   Regularly update your knowledge and skills, particularly in terms of legislation, ethics and best practices. Training courses also raise awareness of legal risks and how to prevent them.

Professional ethics

Beyond legal obligations, professional ethics guide caregivers' actions towards respectful, humane and responsible practice. This implies :

- **Beneficence**: Acting in the patient's interest, promoting well-being and preventing harm.

- **Non-maleficence**: Avoid causing harm to the patient, whether by action or omission.
- **Justice**: Treat all patients fairly, without discrimination, and ensure a fair distribution of resources.
- **Autonomy**: Respecting patients' right to make their own decisions, promoting their autonomy and participation in care.

Relations with families and friends

- Empathetic communication

Empathic communication is an essential skill for geriatric caregivers, enabling them to establish a relationship of trust with the elderly, understand their deepest needs and respond appropriately to their expectations. Empathy is the ability to put oneself in another's shoes, to feel their emotions while maintaining a certain professional distance. In the context of caring for the elderly, who are often faced with health problems, loneliness or loss of autonomy, empathy plays a crucial role in their well-being and quality of life.

The principles of empathic communication

1. **Active listening**: Active listening is the basis of empathic communication. It involves paying full attention to the interlocutor, being fully present in the exchange. This involves concentrating on the patient's words, not interrupting, and showing through non-verbal cues (nodding, looking attentively) that you are following what he or she is saying.

2. **Respect and consideration**: Treating each patient with respect, without judgment or prejudice, is fundamental. This means recognizing each person's dignity, values, beliefs and life history. Unconditional positive consideration fosters a climate of trust and openness.

3. **Authenticity**: Being sincere and authentic in your exchanges builds credibility and trust. The caregiver must avoid artificial attitudes or pretences, and express his or her feelings appropriately.

4. **Emotional responsiveness**: Being sensitive to the patient's emotions, whether expressed verbally or non-verbally. This involves perceiving emotional signals, such as sadness, anxiety or anger, and recognizing them in the exchange.

5. **Appropriate response**: Having understood the patient's emotions and needs, the caregiver must respond appropriately. This can be done through comforting words, supportive gestures or concrete actions to help the patient.

Techniques for developing empathic communication

1. **Use appropriate language**: Use simple words, avoid medical jargon and adapt your speech to the patient's level of understanding. This facilitates understanding and shows that you care about the patient's ability to follow the conversation.

2. **Ask open-ended questions**: Encourage patients to express themselves by asking questions that require more than a yes or no answer. For example, "How are you feeling today?" or "Can you tell me about anything that's worrying you?".

3. **Rephrasing**: Repeating in your own words what the patient has just said, to check understanding and show that you are paying attention. For example, "If I've understood correctly, you're concerned about your next medical procedure, right?

4. **Validating feelings**: Recognize and legitimize the patient's emotions. For example, "I understand why this

might frighten you" or "It's normal to feel sad in this situation".

5. **Empathetic silence**: Knowing how to respect moments of silence, which allow the patient to reflect or express difficult emotions. Silence can be a powerful tool for deepening the exchange.

Obstacles to empathic communication

1. **Prejudice and stereotypes**: Preconceived ideas about the elderly can hinder the ability to truly connect with the patient. It's important to be aware of your own prejudices and put them aside.

2. **Language and cultural barriers**: Differences in language or culture can make communication more difficult. The caregiver has to make an effort to understand the patient, possibly by using interpreters or learning about the patient's culture.

3. **Personal emotions**: The caregiver's own emotions, such as stress or fatigue, can interfere with his or her ability to be empathetic. It is important to manage one's emotions and take care of oneself in order to be available for the patient.

4. **Lack of time**: Organizational constraints can limit the amount of time devoted to each patient. However, even short interactions can be empathetic if you are fully present.

The benefits of empathic communication

1. **Improving the caregiver-patient relationship**: Empathetic communication strengthens the bond of trust, facilitates patient collaboration and enhances satisfaction with the care received.

2. **Better understanding of the patient's needs**: By being attentive and empathetic, the caregiver can identify unexpressed needs, anticipate problems and adapt care accordingly.

3. **Reduced anxiety and distress**: Emotional support through empathic communication can ease patients' fears, reduce stress and promote psychological well-being.

4. **Promoting autonomy**: By valuing the patient's feelings and choices, the caregiver encourages autonomy and involvement in health-related decisions.

Putting empathic communication into practice in geriatrics

1. **Adapting to cognitive disorders**: With patients suffering from dementia or cognitive disorders, empathic communication requires adjustments. Using simple phrases, calmly repeating information and being patient are effective strategies.

2. **Dealing with difficult emotions**: Older people may express anger, frustration or sadness. The caregiver must welcome these emotions without taking them personally, and offer appropriate support.

3. **Respecting individual rhythms**: Take the time needed for each patient, respect their pace of speech and don't rush them, even when time is tight.

4. **Family integration**: The family plays an important role in the patient's well-being. Communicating empathetically with loved ones can strengthen support around the patient and improve the quality of care.

Training and development of empathic communication skills

1. **Self-reflection**: Take time to reflect on your own communication practices, identifying strengths and areas for improvement.

2. **Specific training**: Participate in workshops or training courses on empathic communication, active listening or emotion management.

3. **Supervision and feedback**: Ask for feedback from colleagues or superiors and be open to constructive criticism.

4. **Regular practice**: Like all skills, empathic communication improves with practice. Consciously integrate these techniques into everyday professional life.

- Managing expectations and emotions

Managing expectations and emotions is a fundamental aspect of the caregiver's role in geriatrics. The elderly face many challenges associated with aging, such as loss of autonomy, chronic illness, lifestyle changes and sometimes social isolation. These situations can generate a multitude of emotions, from anxiety and sadness to anger and frustration. What's more, patients and their families often have specific expectations regarding the care they receive. The caregiver must therefore be able to skillfully navigate these expectations and emotions to provide quality care.

Understanding the expectations of patients and their families

The expectations of elderly patients and their families can be varied and influenced by several factors:

1. **Care expectations**: Patients wish to receive care adapted to their needs, with particular attention paid to their comfort and dignity. They expect caregivers to be competent, caring and respectful.

2. **Maintaining independence**: Many older people aspire to remain independent for as long as possible. They may have high expectations of their ability to carry out certain daily activities, even if their state of health limits these possibilities.

3. **Communication and information**: Patients and their families expect clear, honest and empathetic communication. They want to be kept informed about care, treatment and changes in their state of health.

4. **Emotional support**: Faced with the challenges of aging, patients seek emotional support. They expect caregivers to listen to their concerns and help them overcome their anxieties.

To meet these expectations, the caregiver must adopt a patient-centered approach, taking the time to understand the patient's specific needs and adapting his or her interventions accordingly. It is essential to create a relationship of trust, based on mutual respect and consideration.

Managing patients' emotions

The elderly can experience intense emotions linked to their condition. The caregiver must be able to recognize these emotions and manage them appropriately:

1. **Acknowledging and accepting emotions**: It's important to acknowledge the patient's feelings without judging them. Whether it's fear, anger or sadness, these emotions are legitimate and deserve to be heard.

2. **Active listening**: Practice active listening by giving the patient your full attention. This involves letting the patient express himself freely, without interruption, and showing empathy.

3. **Emotional validation**: Validate the patient's emotions by expressing sincere understanding. For example, saying "I understand that this may be difficult for you" can help the patient feel understood and supported.

4. **Offer support**: Suggest solutions or activities that can help patients manage their emotions, such as relaxation exercises, talking about pleasant topics or encouraging them to take part in social activities.

5. **Working with the nursing team**: If the patient shows significant signs of emotional distress, it's crucial to inform the care team so that appropriate care can be taken, possibly with the involvement of a psychologist.

Managing unrealistic expectations

Sometimes, patients or their families may have unrealistic expectations regarding care or the evolution of the disease. In such cases, the caregiver must :

1. **Communicate tactfully**: Explain medical realities and limitations related to the patient's condition in a clear and empathetic manner.

2. **Setting realistic goals**: Work with the patient and family to define achievable goals, rewarding even modest progress.

3. **Involving loved ones**: Encouraging family participation in the care plan, while respecting the patient's wishes, can help align expectations.

4. **Be patient**: Understand that accepting limitations can take time and requires ongoing support.

Managing your own emotions

The caregiver is also confronted with his or her own emotions in difficult situations. To maintain a professional relationship and offer the best possible support, they must :

1. **Develop self-awareness**: Recognize your own emotional reactions, whether to stress, frustration or sadness.

2. **Practice emotional regulation**: Learn techniques for managing stress, such as deep breathing, meditation or regular physical activity.

3. **Seek support**: Don't hesitate to share your feelings with colleagues, superiors or mental health professionals.

4. **Avoid burnout**: Balance your professional and personal life, take regular breaks and give yourself time to recharge.

Communication strategies for effective management

Effective communication is the key to managing expectations and emotions:

1. **Clarity and transparency**: Provide precise, understandable information, avoiding medical jargon.

2. **Empathy in communication**: Adapt your verbal and non-verbal language to express compassion and understanding.

3. **Constructive feedback**: Encourage patients to express their feelings and concerns, and respond positively.

4. **Adaptation**: Take into account the patient's cognitive abilities, particularly in the case of memory or attention disorders, by using visual aids or repeating information if necessary.

Promoting autonomy and dignity

Respecting patients' autonomy and dignity is paramount:

1. **Encourage participation**: Involve patients in decisions concerning their care, respecting their choices and preferences.

2. **Valuing remaining abilities**: Focus on what patients can still do, rather than on their limitations, to boost their self-confidence.

3. **Adapt interventions**: Personalize care according to the patient's needs and desires, taking into account his or her life history, culture and values.

- Supporting care decisions

Supporting the elderly in making care decisions is an essential dimension of the caregiver's role in geriatrics. The aim is to support patients in the decision-making process concerning their health, while respecting their autonomy, values and preferences. In a context where the elderly may be confronted with complex medical situations, cognitive limitations or external pressures, the caregiver plays a key role in facilitating understanding, the expression of choices and the implementation of care decisions.

Importance of patient autonomy and choice

Autonomy is a fundamental principle of medical ethics, which recognizes the right of each individual to make informed decisions about his or her own health. For the elderly, preserving this autonomy is crucial to maintaining their dignity, self-esteem and quality of life. The caregiver must ensure that the patient is at the center of the decision-making process, taking into account his or her abilities, wishes and personal context.

The caregiver's role in decision support

1. **Facilitating comprehension**

   The caregiver can help the patient understand medical information by:

   - **Simplifying language**: Use accessible words, avoid medical jargon and explain complex terms.
   - **Using visual aids**: diagrams, illustrations or written documents can help clarify explanations.
   - **Answering questions**: Encourage patients to express their questions, and answer them with patience and clarity.

2. **Assessment of decision-making ability**

   It is important to recognize whether the patient is capable of making informed decisions. In the event of cognitive impairment or confusion, the caregiver must :

   - **Observe signs of disorientation**: memory difficulties, language disorders, inattention.
   - **Inform the care team**: Report these observations for further medical evaluation.
   - **Adapt communication**: use simple sentences, repeat information if necessary, check understanding.

3. **Emotional support**

   Making decisions about one's health can be a source of anxiety and stress for the patient. The caregiver must :

   - **Offer a reassuring presence**: Be available, show empathy and understanding.

- **Validate emotions**: Acknowledge the patient's feelings, be they fear, doubt or frustration.
- **Encourage expression**: Invite patients to share their concerns, hopes and expectations.

4. **Promoting active participation**

   To reinforce the patient's involvement in care decisions, the caregiver can:

   - **Involve the patient in discussions**: Encourage them to attend meetings with the care team or ask questions during consultations.
   - **Respecting patients' choices**: Even if patients' decisions differ from medical recommendations, it is essential to respect their wishes, as long as they are capable of making their own decisions.
   - **Promote autonomy**: Offer options, let the patient choose between different alternatives when they exist.

Working with family and friends

The family often plays an important role in care decisions for the elderly. The caregiver must:

1. **Facilitating communication**

   - **Mediating**: Helping to clarify information between patient, family and care team.
   - **Ensuring that the patient's wishes are heard**: Make sure that the patient's voice is at the center of discussions, especially in the case of family disagreements.

2. Respect confidentiality and consent

- **Protect personal information**: share information with family only with the patient's consent.
- **Inform about the role of the trusted support person**: If the patient so wishes, he or she can designate a trusted support person to accompany him or her in making decisions.

Taking account of advance directives

Advance directives are written documents in which a person expresses his or her wishes concerning the medical care he or she wishes to receive or not receive if he or she is no longer able to communicate his or her decisions. The caregiver must:

1. Knowing about directives

- **Find out**: Check whether the patient has written advance directives and where they are kept.
- **Respecting wishes**: Ensuring that directives are taken into account when making care decisions.

2. Raising patient awareness

- **Inform about the importance of directives**: Explain to patients the usefulness of writing directives to ensure that their future wishes are respected.
- **Referring to resources**: If the patient wants to find out more, help him or her contact a competent professional (doctor, social worker, etc.).

Managing situations of refusal of care

The patient may refuse a proposed treatment or intervention. The caregiver must then :

1. **Understanding the reasons for refusal**

    - **Dialogue with the patient**: Try to understand his or her motivations, whether they are linked to fears, beliefs or past experiences.
    - **Identify barriers**: Perhaps the patient has unexpressed fears or incomplete information.

2. **Informing the care team**

    - **Passing on information**: Communicate the refusal and associated reasons to the nurse or doctor so that they can deal with the situation appropriately.
    - **Participate in the search for solutions**: Collaborate to find alternatives or adapt the care plan.

Adapting to the patient's cognitive abilities

For patients with cognitive disorders, support in making care decisions requires adjustments:

1. **Simplified information**

    - **Use appropriate media**: pictures, pictograms, concrete objects to illustrate explanations.
    - **Repeat and reformulate**: Present information several times, using different words.

2. **Respecting the level of understanding**

    - **Assess the patient's capacity to consent**: If the patient is no longer able to make informed decisions, it's important to follow legal procedures, such as appointing a guardian or a support person.

Ethics and deontology in decision support

The caregiver must act in accordance with ethical principles:

1. **Charity**

    - **Act in the patient's interest**: Propose actions to improve health and well-being.

2. **Non-maleficence**

    - **Do no harm**: Refrain from imposing decisions or interventions not desired by the patient.

3. **Justice**

    - **Ensuring equity**: offering the same level of attention and respect to all patients, without discrimination.

4. **Respect for autonomy**

    - **Valuing the patient's ability to decide**: Even in the presence of limitations, seek to involve the patient as much as possible.

Training and professional development

To be effective in supporting care decisions, the caregiver must :

1. **Communication training**

    - **Improve your skills**: Take part in training courses on therapeutic communication, active listening and managing difficult situations.

2. **Know the legal aspects**

    ◦ **Master patients' rights**: Inform about informed consent, advance directives and the role of the trusted support person.

3. **Developing cultural awareness**

    ◦ **Understand cultural influences**: Values and beliefs can influence care decisions. Be open and respectful of cultural differences.

Chapter 3

Basic geriatric care

Hygiene and Patient Comfort

- Adapted grooming techniques

Toileting is an essential part of caring for the elderly. It is not limited to bodily hygiene, but has a social, psychological and relational dimension. For geriatric caregivers, mastering appropriate grooming techniques is essential to ensure the comfort, safety and well-being of patients, while respecting their dignity and autonomy. In a context where the elderly may have physical, cognitive or sensory limitations, it is essential to adapt care to meet their specific needs.

The importance of adapted grooming in geriatrics

Daily grooming contributes to :

- **Maintain personal hygiene**: prevent infections, skin irritations and unpleasant odors.
- **Preserving dignity and self-esteem**: Feeling clean and cared for enhances psychological well-being.
- **Promote physical comfort**: relieve discomfort caused by perspiration, secretions or incontinence.
- **Monitor health**: enable the caregiver to detect abnormal skin signs (bedsores, erythema, wounds).
- **Creating a relationship**: Toileting is a privileged moment for exchange and communication.

General principles for adapted grooming

1. **Respecting dignity and privacy**
   It is essential to preserve the patient's privacy by closing the door, using screens and covering unwashed parts of the body with a towel. The caregiver must explain every gesture, ask for consent before starting, and respect the patient's habits and preferences.

2. **Promoting autonomy**
   Encourage patients to participate in toileting according

to their abilities. This can reinforce autonomy and self-esteem. The caregiver must adapt his or her assistance, neither too much to avoid infantilizing the patient, nor too little to avoid fatigue or the risk of falling.

3. **Safety and comfort**
   Ensure a safe environment by checking water temperature, avoiding slippery surfaces and using appropriate equipment (grab bars, shower seats). Patient comfort is paramount: pleasant room temperature, gentle gestures, respect for the patient's rhythm.

4. **Appropriate communication**
   Use clear language, adapted to the patient's level of understanding. Be attentive to non-verbal signs, especially in patients with cognitive disorders, to detect possible discomfort or refusal.

Specific techniques for different contexts

1. **Washbasin toilet**

   - **Preparing equipment**: Gather everything you need (washcloths, mild soap, towels, clean clothes) to avoid back-and-forth movements and keep the patient warm.
   - **Patient set-up**: Make sure the patient is comfortably seated in a secure chair, with supports if necessary.
   - **Active participation**: Encourage patients to wash their face, hands and upper body if they are able, with guidance and physical support if necessary.
   - **Targeted assistance**: Help in hard-to-reach areas or if the patient shows signs of fatigue.

2. **Toilet in bed**

    - **Indications** : For patients who are bedridden, tired or at risk of falling.
    - **Organization**: develop a methodology to avoid excessive patient handling and reduce discomfort.
    - **Technology**:
        - **Hand hygiene**: caregivers must wash their hands before and after washing.
        - **Sequencing**: Start with face, then upper body, arms, hands, chest, abdomen, legs, feet, back, private parts.
        - **Protecting bedding**: Use undersheets to avoid wetting the bed.
        - **Respect for privacy**: uncover only the part of the body to be washed.
        - **Gentle mobilization**: Carefully turn the patient, following handling techniques to avoid pain and trauma.

3. **Toilet in the shower or bath**

    - **Pre-assessment**: Check that the patient can be moved safely to the bathroom.
    - **Safety** :
        - **Adapted equipment**: Shower seat, non-slip mat, grab bars.
        - **Constant supervision**: Never leave the patient alone if his balance is precarious.
    - **Comfort** :
        - **Water temperature**: Check with a thermometer or wrist test (approx. 37°C).
        - **Warm atmosphere**: Heat the room if necessary.

- **Patient participation**: Encourage the patient to wash, intervening in difficult areas or if fatigue occurs.

Adaptations for patients with specific disorders

1. **Patients with cognitive disorders (dementia, Alzheimer's)**

   - **Calm, reassuring approach**: Introduce yourself, explain each step, use a gentle tone.
   - **Consistent routine**: Maintain regular grooming schedules to establish a sense of security.
   - **Sensory stimulation**: Use pleasantly scented products and soft music to make the moment pleasant.
   - **Respecting refusal**: If the patient refuses the toilet, do not force it. Offer to come back later or adapt the method.

2. **Patients with reduced mobility**

   - **Use of technical aids**: patient lifts, transfer belts, sliding boards.
   - **Preventing falls**: Make sure the floor is dry and that the patient is wearing non-slip slippers.
   - **Ergonomic positioning**: Adapt the height of the bed or chair to avoid unnecessary effort.

3. **Incontinent patients**

   - **Rigorous intimate hygiene**: Gently cleanse the perineal area with suitable products and dry thoroughly to prevent irritation.
   - **Skin protection**: Apply barrier creams if necessary.
   - **Discreet management**: Approach the situation tactfully to preserve the patient's dignity.

4. **Patients with wounds or pressure sores**
    - **Washing precautions**: Avoid rubbing fragile areas, use gentle products.
    - **Monitoring**: Take advantage of washing to inspect the skin, and report any abnormalities to the care team.
    - **Positioning**: Alternate positions to reduce pressure on high-risk areas.

Relational aspects of grooming

- **Creating a climate of trust**: Establishing a relationship based on respect, listening and caring.
- **Personalization**: Take into account patient habits (product preferences, order of steps, rituals).
- **Communication**: Talk to the patient, even if he or she doesn't respond, to maintain the social link.
- **Observation**: Take advantage of this special moment to detect signs of discomfort, pain or isolation.

Infection prevention

- **Hand hygiene**: Before and after each treatment, use a hydroalcoholic solution or wash hands with soap and water.
- **Wearing gloves** : For intimate hygiene or if the patient has skin lesions.
- **Equipment maintenance**: Clean and disinfect equipment after use.
- **Linen management**: Regularly change towels, washcloths and clothes.

Training and skills updating

The caregiver must undergo regular training to :

- **New techniques**: Innovations in technical aids, adapted products, care protocols.
- **Updating knowledge**: hygiene rules, prevention of nosocomial infections, management of cognitive disorders.
- **Developing interpersonal skills**: non-verbal communication, patient-centered approach, managing difficult situations.

- Skin care and pressure sore prevention

The skin is the largest organ in the human body, and plays an essential role in protection against external aggression, temperature regulation and sensory perception. In the elderly, the skin undergoes physiological changes that make it more vulnerable to damage, particularly pressure sores. Preventing pressure sores is a priority in geriatrics, as they can have serious consequences for patients' health and quality of life. The caregiver plays a central role in skin care and the implementation of preventive measures.

Understanding age-related skin changes

As we age, our skin undergoes several changes:

1. **Thinner epidermis and dermis**: skin becomes thinner, reducing its ability to resist mechanical trauma.

2. **Decreased elasticity**: collagen and elastin production are reduced, making skin less supple and more fragile.

3. **Skin dryness**: Reduced sebum and sweat production leads to dry skin, which can cause itching and cracking.

4. **Reduced vascularity**: Cutaneous blood flow is reduced, delaying healing and response to lesions.

5. **Impaired sensory perception**: Sensitivity to touch, pressure and pain may be reduced, limiting the

perception of discomfort associated with prolonged pressure.

Factors contributing to the development of pressure sores

Pressure sores are skin lesions resulting from prolonged pressure on an area of the body, leading to tissue ischemia and necrosis. Several factors increase the risk of pressure sores in the elderly:

1. **Immobility**: Reduced mobility, due to neurological conditions, fractures or general weakness, encourages continuous pressure on certain areas.

2. **Incontinence**: skin exposure to moisture and irritants in urine and feces weakens the epidermis.

3. **Malnutrition and dehydration**: Insufficient intake of essential nutrients weakens the skin and delays healing.

4. **Chronic pathologies**: Diabetes, vascular or neurological diseases alter sensitivity and vascularization, increasing the risk of lesions.

5. **Advanced age**: Skin changes linked to aging accentuate the fragility of the skin.

Pressure sore prevention strategies

Prevention is based on a multidisciplinary approach and the rigorous application of specific measures:

1. **Risk assessment**: Use of assessment tools such as the Norton or Braden scales to identify patients at risk and adapt interventions.

2. **Regular mobilization**: Change the patient's position frequently, at least every two hours, to reduce pressure on at-risk areas.

3. **Use of suitable supports**: anti-bedsore mattresses, special cushions to distribute pressure and reduce excessive pressure points.

4. **Appropriate hygiene care**: Keep skin clean and dry, use mild, moisturizing products to preserve skin integrity.

5. **Adequate nutrition**: Ensure an adequate supply of proteins, vitamins and minerals to promote skin health and healing.

6. **Sufficient hydration**: Encourage regular fluid intake to maintain skin elasticity.

7. **Incontinence management**: Use absorbent pads, change soiled pads frequently, apply skin barriers to protect the skin.

8. **Patient and family education**: Inform about pressure sore risks and preventive measures to encourage collaboration.

The role of the caregiver in skin care and pressure sore prevention

The caregiver is at the forefront of observing, preventing and reporting signs of skin deterioration:

1. **Careful observation of the skin**

    - **Daily inspection**: Examine at-risk areas when washing or changing clothes, especially points of support (heels, sacrum, hips, elbows, shoulder blades).
    - **Detection of early signs**: persistent redness, induration, local heat, edema or pain.

2. **Mobilization and positioning**

    - **Change of position**: Help the patient turn regularly, use mobilization techniques that are safe for both patient and caregiver.
    - **Body alignment**: Ensure a comfortable position, avoiding folds in sheets or clothing which can create pressure points.

3. **Hygiene care and skin hydration**

    - **Use appropriate products**: Choose mild, fragrance-free soaps and moisturizing lotions to prevent skin dryness.
    - **Gentle technique**: Avoid excessive friction when washing or drying, gently dab the skin.

4. **Humidity management**

    - **Incontinence management**: Promptly change soiled pads, clean skin thoroughly, apply barrier creams.
    - **Control perspiration**: Dress the patient in light, breathable, natural fabrics.

5. **Using prevention media**

    - **Correct installation of devices**: Place cushions, wedges or specialized mattresses correctly to maximize their effectiveness.
    - **Regular checks**: ensure equipment is in good condition, report any faults or wear to the care team.

6. **Encouraging mobility**

    ○ **Stimulation of autonomy**: Encourage patients to perform even minimal movements to promote blood circulation.
    ○ **Adapted activities**: Suggest simple exercises, in collaboration with physiotherapists, to maintain joint mobility.

7. **Communication with the care team**

    ○ **Rapid reporting**: Immediately inform the nurse or doctor if alarming signs are detected.
    ○ **Participation in meetings**: Contribute to discussions on the care plan, share observations and propose solutions.

Specific skin care techniques

1. **Adapted toilet**

    ○ **Appropriate frequency**: Adapt the frequency of cleansing to the patient's condition, avoiding over-frequent baths which can dry out the skin.
    ○ **Water temperature**: Use lukewarm water to avoid vasoconstriction or excessive dilation of skin vessels.

2. **Skin hydration**

    ○ **Regular application of creams**: Use emollients after washing to maintain hydration.
    ○ **Choice of products**: Choose hypoallergenic products, without colorants or perfumes.

3. **Light massage**

    ○ **Stimulate circulation**: Gently massage around at-risk areas to encourage blood flow, avoiding direct massage of red or already damaged areas.

4. **Protection against trauma**

    ○ **Handling precautions**: Avoid pulling or rubbing the skin, and lift the patient gently during transfers.
    ○ **Preventing friction and shearing** : Use sliding sheets or appropriate techniques to reduce shearing forces.

Monitoring and documentation

- **Keeping accurate records**: recording observations, procedures carried out and changes in the patient's skin condition.
- **Use of assessment tools**: employ pressure sore monitoring grids, enabling standardized assessment and regular follow-up.

Patient and family education

- **Risk awareness**: Explain pressure sore risk factors and the importance of preventive measures.
- **Involvement in care**: Encourage the patient and family to participate in position changes, exercises or skin monitoring.
- **Practical advice**: Provide recommendations on diet, hydration and the use of home equipment.

Interprofessional collaboration

- **Teamwork**: Working with nurses, doctors, physiotherapists, dieticians and occupational therapists to provide comprehensive care.
- **Protocol updates**: Participate in training and meetings to keep abreast of best practices and institutional protocols.

- Installation and refurbishment of healthcare bed

The healthcare bed is a central element in the care of patients in hospitals, residential care facilities for the dependent elderly (EHPAD) or at home. It's not just functional furniture, but an essential tool for ensuring patient comfort, safety and well-being. Setting up and refurbishing a healthcare bed is a crucial task for the caregiver, who must master the appropriate techniques while complying with hygiene and safety protocols. Although often seen as a routine task, it requires special attention to prevent the risk of infection, falls or patient discomfort.

The importance of the healthcare bed in patient care

The medical bed offers specific features adapted to patients' needs:

1. **Height adjustment**: Facilitates care by nursing staff and patient transfers.
2. **Back and leg adjustment**: Adjusts patient position for comfort, breathing, digestion and pressure sore prevention.
3. **Side rails**: Prevent falls, secure the patient.
4. **Wheels with brakes**: Mobility of the bed to facilitate cleaning or patient movement, while ensuring stability once the brakes are activated.

Proper installation and refurbishment of the healthcare bed helps to :

- **Ensuring patient comfort**: A clean, well-made bed, adapted to the patient's needs, enhances well-being.
- **Prevent infections**: Compliance with hygiene protocols limits the risk of cross-contamination.
- **Facilitating care**: A well-organized bed enables the caregiver to intervene effectively.
- **Prevent accidents**: A safe installation reduces the risk of falls or injury.

Preparation prior to bed installation or refurbishment

1. **Hand hygiene**: Before any handling, the caregiver must perform rigorous hand hygiene using a hydroalcoholic solution, or by washing with soap if hands are soiled.

2. **Materials required**:
   - Clean fitted sheet
   - Absorbent undersheet or mattress protector
   - Flat sheet
   - Blanket or comforter
   - Pillowcase
   - Pillow(s) and optional bolster
   - Accessories: positioning cushions, anti-bedsore supports
   - Bag for dirty laundry

3. **Checking equipment condition** :
   - Check that the bed is in good condition and that the mechanisms are working properly.
   - Check that the mattress is intact, with no tears or stains.
   - Make sure wheel brakes are operational.

4. **Environmental safety** :
    - Clear the space around the bed to facilitate movement.
    - Make sure the floor is dry to avoid the risk of slipping.

Vacuum bed repair technique

When the patient is not in bed, refurbishment is easier:

1. **Bed positioning** :
    - **Height**: Set the bed at an ergonomic height to avoid unnecessary effort and prevent musculoskeletal disorders.
    - **Brakes**: Check that the brakes are engaged to stabilize the bed.

2. **Soiled linen removal** :
    - Unfold the bed by successively removing the blanket, flat sheet, draw sheet and fitted sheet.
    - Roll soiled linen inwards to contain soiling.
    - Place soiled linen directly into the bag provided, without placing it on the floor or on a clean surface.

3. **Mattress cleaning** :
    - If necessary, clean the mattress with a suitable disinfectant, respecting the recommended contact times.
    - Allow mattress to dry before making up the bed.

4. **Installation of clean linen** :

    - **Fitted sheet**: Stretch the fitted sheet well to avoid creases, which can be uncomfortable for the patient and encourage pressure sores.
    - **Absorbent underpad**: Place the underpad in the center of the bed, where the patient's pelvis is located, to protect the mattress from any leaks.
    - **Flat sheet**: Lay the flat sheet on the bed, leaving enough length on each side.
    - **Blanket or comforter**: Place the blanket or comforter on the flat sheet.
    - **Edge**: create a hospital fold at the foot of the bed to hold the sheet and blanket in place, while leaving room for the patient's feet.
    - **Pillow(s)**: Put the pillow in its case and place it at the head of the bed.

Technique for restoring an occupied bed

When the patient is bedridden and cannot leave the bed, extra care is needed to ensure comfort and safety.

1. **Communication with the patient** :

    - **Explanation**: Inform the patient of the procedure, obtain his consent and reassure him.
    - **Participation**: Encouraging patients to participate to the best of their ability, thereby promoting their autonomy and well-being.

2. **Preparation**:

    - **Equipment on hand**: Keep all necessary equipment close at hand to avoid leaving the patient alone.

- **Safety**: Make sure side rails are in place on the opposite side of the machine from where you are working, to prevent falls.

3. **Step-by-step technique** :

    - **Right side** :
        - Help the patient to turn onto his left side, gently, supporting the necessary body parts.
        - Roll the dirty linen along the length of the bed to the center, bringing it closer to the patient.
        - Place the clean fitted sheet on the exposed part of the mattress, securing it at the corners.
        - Fold unused clean linen under rolled dirty linen.

    - **Left side** :
        - Help the patient turn onto his right side, passing over the roll of dirty and clean linen.
        - Remove soiled linen and place in laundry bag.
        - Unfold the clean fitted sheet over the rest of the mattress and secure.
        - Help the patient to reposition comfortably on his or her back.

    - **Finalization** :
        - Install the absorbent underpad using the same technique if necessary.

- Lay out the flat sheet, blanket or comforter, making sure the patient is covered and comfortable.
- Adjust the pillow and make sure the patient is comfortable.

4. **Special precautions** :

   - **Pain prevention**: Handle the patient gently, avoiding sudden movements.
   - **Observation**: Take advantage of the dressing process to observe the patient's skin condition, especially areas at risk of pressure sores.
   - **Hygiene**: Change gloves if necessary, observe hygiene rules to prevent infection.

Adaptations for specific patients

1. **Disabled or dependent patients**:

   - **Use of technical aids**: patient lifts, sliding sheets to facilitate movement without excessive effort.
   - **Working in pairs**: Working with a colleague to ensure patient and caregiver safety.

2. **Restless or confused patients**:

   - **Soothing approach**: Speak calmly, explain every gesture, respect the patient's rhythm.
   - **Increased safety**: Keep side rails in place, watch out for unexpected movements.

3. **Patients with medical devices** :

   - **Caution with probes and catheters**: Avoid pulling or pinching devices when handling linen.
   - **Coordination with the team**: If necessary, enlist the nurse's help to handle devices safely.

Hygiene and infection control

1. **Dirty linen management** :
   - **Sorting**: Separate biologically soiled linen from unsoiled linen according to protocols.
   - **Transport**: Use suitable bags, close bags before moving them, avoid placing them on the ground.

2. **Hand hygiene** :
   - **Frequency**: Before and after bed-making, after handling soiled linen.
   - **Technique**: Follow recommendations for effective washing or rubbing with hydroalcoholic solution.

3. **Equipment disinfection** :
   - **Contact surfaces**: Clean side gates, remote controls and handles after refurbishment if necessary.
   - **Suitable products**: Use disinfectants that comply with institutional protocols.

Ergonomics and prevention of musculoskeletal disorders

1. **Proper posture** :
   - **Straight back**: Avoid leaning forward, bend your knees to reach the lower parts of the bed.
   - **Proximity**: Move closer to the bed to limit arm extension.

2. **Use of force** :
   - **Firm footing**: Position yourself stably with your feet hip-width apart.

- **Fluid movements**: Avoid sudden movements or twisting of the trunk.

Patient relations and well-being

1. **Positive communication**:
   - **Empathy**: listening to the patient's feelings, responding to his or her needs.
   - **Respect**: Maintain a benevolent attitude, avoid unprofessional conversations during refurbishment.

2. **Post-refinement comfort** :
   - **Checking**: Make sure the patient is comfortable and that nothing is in the way (folds, objects left in the bed).
   - **Accessibility**: Place call bell, glass of water and personal belongings within easy reach.

Nutrition and hydration

- Specific nutritional requirements

Nutrition plays a fundamental role in maintaining the health, well-being and quality of life of the elderly. As people age, their nutritional needs evolve, and many factors can influence their nutritional status. In geriatrics, it is essential to understand these specific needs in order to prevent undernutrition, micronutritional deficiencies and associated complications. The caregiver, by virtue of his or her proximity to patients, is in a privileged position to observe, prevent and intervene with regard to nutrition.

Physiological changes affecting nutrition in the elderly

With age, the body undergoes several physiological changes that influence nutritional requirements:

1. **Decreased muscle mass**: sarcopenia, a progressive loss of muscle mass and strength, can affect mobility and increase the risk of falls.

2. **Reduced basal metabolic** rate: Metabolism slows down, which may lead to a reduction in caloric requirements, but essential nutrient requirements remain unchanged or increase.

3. **Altered senses**: Decreased sense of taste and smell can reduce appetite and the pleasure of eating, leading to reduced food consumption.

4. **Dental and digestive problems**: Chewing difficulties, dry mouth, swallowing disorders (dysphagia) and gastrointestinal problems can limit food intake.

5. **Changes in nutrient absorption**: The absorption of certain nutrients, such as vitamin B12, calcium and vitamin D, may be reduced due to changes in the digestive system.

Specific nutritional needs of the elderly

1. **Protein**: Seniors need sufficient protein intake to maintain muscle mass and immune function. A slightly higher protein intake is recommended than for younger adults, with a preference for high-quality protein sources.

2. **Energy (calories)**: Although the basal metabolic rate declines, it's important to consume enough calories to meet energy needs, especially during illness or convalescence.

3. **Dietary fiber**: Adequate fiber intake is essential to prevent constipation, improve digestive health and regulate blood sugar levels.

4. **Hydration**: Elderly people are more likely to become dehydrated due to a reduced sensation of thirst. Regular hydration is crucial to the body's proper functioning.

5. **Vitamins and minerals** :

    - **Vitamin D**: Essential for bone health and immune function. Skin synthesis of vitamin D declines with age, requiring dietary intake or supplementation.

    - **Calcium**: Essential for maintaining bone density and preventing osteoporosis.

    - **Vitamin B12**: Important for nerve function and red blood cell production. Absorption may be reduced in the elderly.

    - **Iron**: Necessary to prevent anemia, but excess can be harmful.

    - **Zinc**: Plays a role in healing, immune function and taste.

Factors influencing the nutritional status of the elderly

1. **Socio-economic factors**: Limited financial resources can restrict access to a variety of quality foods.

2. **Social isolation**: Loneliness can reduce the desire to prepare meals and eat, leading to a reduction in food intake.

3. **Cognitive disorders**: Dementia or Alzheimer's disease can lead to forgetting meals or eating inappropriately.

4. **Polypharmacy**: Taking multiple medications can affect appetite, taste, digestion or nutrient absorption.

5. **Depression**: Mood disorders can reduce appetite and interest in food.

Strategies to meet specific nutritional needs

1. **Balanced and varied diet**: Offer meals that cover all food groups, with an emphasis on lean proteins, fruit, vegetables, whole grains and dairy products.

2. **Meal enrichment**: Adding calories and nutrients to foods (e.g. adding powdered milk to soups, using olive oil, incorporating eggs into purees) to increase nutritional density without increasing volume.

3. **Adapted textures**: In the event of chewing or swallowing difficulties, adapt the texture of food (minced, blended, thickened liquids) to facilitate ingestion while preserving taste pleasure.

4. **Frequent small meals**: Offer snacks between meals to increase calorie intake and avoid rapid satiety.

5. **Regular hydration**: Encourage fluid intake throughout the day, by offering water, herbal teas, broths or diluted fruit juices.

6. **Pleasant atmosphere**: Create a friendly environment for meals, encouraging social interaction, careful presentation of dishes and a relaxed atmosphere.

7. **Supplementation if required**: Under medical supervision, supplements of specific vitamins, minerals or nutrients may be prescribed.

8. **Respecting food preferences**: Take into account the patient's tastes, cultural habits and dietary restrictions to increase the acceptability of meals.

The caregiver's role in nutritional management

1. **Observation and detection of signs of undernutrition** :

    - Monitor weight changes.
    - Note changes in appetite or food refusal.
    - Observe physical signs such as fatigue, muscle weakness and skin disorders.

2. **Food assistance** :

    - Assist patients with meals, if necessary, while respecting their autonomy.
    - Encourage patients to eat, without rushing them, by adopting a benevolent attitude.

3. **Communication with the care team** :

    - Report eating, swallowing or dental problems to the nurse or doctor.
    - Participate in follow-up meetings to adapt the nutritional care plan.

4. **Education and awareness** :

    - Inform patients about the importance of a balanced diet.
    - Encourage family and friends to participate and support the patient's eating habits.

5. **Adapting to the environment** :
    - Make sure the patient is comfortable to eat.
    - Ensure that utensils are suitable (ergonomic cutlery, spill-proof glasses).

6. **Preventing dehydration**:
    - Offer drinks on a regular basis, even in the absence of demand.
    - Watch for signs of dehydration: dry mouth, confusion, hypotension.

Special cases and considerations

1. **Diabetes**: Adapt your diet to control blood sugar levels, in collaboration with your dietician and doctor.

2. **Renal insufficiency**: Limit certain nutrients such as sodium, potassium or protein according to medical recommendations.

3. **Food allergies or intolerances**: Identify foods to avoid and suggest safe alternatives.

4. **Cultural or religious diets**: Respect dietary restrictions linked to the patient's beliefs.

- Help with meals

Assisting with meals is an essential part of the caregiver's role in geriatrics. Meals are not only a time for nutrition, but also an opportunity for socialization, pleasure and maintaining autonomy for the elderly. However, with advancing age, many obstacles can hinder seniors' ability to eat properly, whether physical, cognitive or emotional. The caregiver therefore plays a crucial role in supporting patients at this key moment of the day, looking after their nutritional needs, safety and overall well-being.

The challenges of feeding the elderly

Several factors can complicate mealtimes for seniors:

1. **Swallowing disorders (dysphagia)**: Difficulty swallowing can lead to the risk of a false route or choking, requiring adaptation of food texture and increased monitoring.

2. **Reduced appetite**: Linked to physiological changes, drug side-effects or psychological disorders such as depression, loss of appetite can lead to undernutrition.

3. **Dental problems**: Missing teeth, unsuitable dentures or mouth pain can make chewing difficult.

4. **Cognitive disorders**: Illnesses such as dementia or Alzheimer's disease can lead to confusion when eating, difficulty using cutlery or recognizing food.

5. **Physical limitations**: Reduced muscle strength, tremors or impaired coordination can hamper the ability to feed oneself independently.

6. **Social isolation**: Eating alone can reduce the pleasure of eating, thus diminishing the desire to eat.

The caregiver's role in assisting with meals

The caregiver intervenes at several levels to facilitate the feeding of the elderly:

1. **Preparing the environment**
   - **Pleasant atmosphere**: Create a friendly atmosphere by carefully setting the table, avoiding distractions such as noise or bustle.
   - **Patient comfort**: Make sure the patient is comfortable, with adequate back support, feet on

the floor or on a footrest, and an upright sitting position to facilitate swallowing.
- **Accessibility**: Place cutlery, glasses and plates within easy reach, taking into account the patient's motor limitations.

2. Adapting meals

- **Modified textures**: Offer chopped, blended or thickened foods in cases of dysphagia, following the recommendations of the doctor or dietician.
- **Small, frequent portions**: Offer several small meals throughout the day if the patient has a reduced appetite.
- **Food preferences**: Take into account tastes, cultural habits and dietary restrictions to increase palatability.

3. Meal assistance

- **Encouraging autonomy**: Encourage patients to feed themselves whenever possible, by providing appropriate cutlery (ergonomic handles, rimmed plates).
- **Direct assistance**: If necessary, help the patient by spoon-feeding, taking care to respect the patient's rhythm and avoiding pressure.
- **Communication**: Explain what's being served, stimulate the senses by describing flavors and aromas to whet the appetite.

4. Surveillance and security

- **Careful observation**: Watch for signs of difficulty, such as coughing, voice changes or expressions of discomfort.

- **False-route prevention**: Ensure proper positioning, adapt feeding speed, check that mouth is empty before each new mouthful.
- **React appropriately in the event of a problem**: Know the first-aid measures to take in the event of choking, and immediately alert the health-care team if necessary.

5. **Emotional and social support**

   - **Positive interaction**: Engage in conversation, listen to the patient, share pleasant moments to make the meal more convivial.
   - **Respect and dignity**: Avoid infantilization, respect food refusals, pay attention to non-verbal signals.

Techniques and tips to make eating easier

1. **Use of technical aids**

   - **Specialized cutlery**: Curved forks and spoons, beakers, non-slip plates.
   - **Food thickeners**: For liquids, to reduce the risk of false ejection.

2. **Appetite stimulation**

   - **Vary menus**: Offer a variety of dishes to avoid monotony.
   - **Careful presentation**: Visually appetizing dishes can encourage people to eat.
   - **Adapted seasonings**: Use herbs and spices to enhance flavours, especially if the sense of taste is impaired.

3. **Managing cognitive disorders**

    ○ **Simplifying the environment**: Reduce disruptive elements on the table, use contrasting crockery to make it easier to distinguish foods.
    ○ **Guidance**: Show gestures, guide the patient's hand if necessary, use simple phrases to give instructions.

4. **Respect for individual rhythms**

    ○ **Sufficient time**: Let patients eat at their own pace, avoid rushing them.
    ○ **Adapting schedules**: Offer meals at times when the patient is most willing to eat.

Collaboration with the care team and family

1. **Information transmission**

    ○ **Observations**: Note quantities eaten, difficulties encountered, changes in appetite.
    ○ **Communication**: Inform the nurse, doctor or dietician of nutritional concerns to adjust the care plan.

2. **Family education and support**

    ○ **Practical advice**: share tips with your family to make mealtimes easier at home.
    ○ **Involvement**: Encourage loved ones to take part in meals, which can strengthen the emotional bond and stimulate the patient's appetite.

Preventing undernutrition and dehydration

Undernutrition is a major risk for the elderly, with serious consequences such as reduced immune defenses, increased risk of bedsores and loss of autonomy. The caregiver must therefore be attentive to :

- **Signs of undernutrition**: involuntary weight loss, clothing becoming too loose, excessive fatigue, muscle wasting.
- **Sufficient water intake**: Offer drinks regularly, even when thirst is not expressed, giving preference to water, herbal teas or fruit juices.

Ethical and respectful approach

1. **Consent and choice**

    - **Respect refusals**: If the patient refuses to eat, it's important to understand the reasons without forcing them, and to offer alternatives later.
    - **Involvement in decision-making**: Involve patients in menu selection wherever possible.

2. **Preserving dignity**

    - **Discretion**: Avoid making negative comments about the patient's eating habits.
    - **Hygiene**: Ensure that the patient is clean before and after meals, and discreetly clean up any soiling.

Training and skills development

The caregiver must undergo regular training to :

- **Eating disorders**: understanding the causes, manifestations and means of intervention.
- **Mastering management techniques**: safe gestures, use of technical aids, adapting to different types of dysphagia.

- **Communication awareness**: Developing verbal and non-verbal communication skills, especially with patients with cognitive disorders.

- Monitoring intake and swallowing disorders

Monitoring food intake and swallowing disorders is an essential component of geriatric care for the elderly. With advancing age, many patients find it difficult to eat properly, which can lead to serious complications such as undernutrition, dehydration and lung infections linked to false routes. The caregiver plays a crucial role in identifying, monitoring and managing these problems, helping to maintain patients' health and well-being.

Understanding swallowing disorders

Swallowing is a complex process involving the coordination of several muscles and nerves. In the elderly, this mechanism can be impaired by various factors:

1. **Physiological changes**: Natural aging leads to reduced muscle strength and coordination, affecting chewing and swallowing.

2. **Neurological pathologies**: Diseases such as stroke, Parkinson's disease or dementia can disrupt neuromuscular control of swallowing.

3. **Local conditions**: Dental problems, dry mouth or oropharyngeal infections can complicate the act of eating.

4. **Drug side effects**: Some drugs can reduce salivation or affect muscle tone, exacerbating swallowing difficulties.

Importance of monitoring food and water intake

Adequate nutritional intake is vital for :

- **Maintain muscle mass**: prevent sarcopenia and preserve functional autonomy.
- **Support the immune system**: Reduce the risk of infection and promote healing.
- **Ensure adequate hydration**: Prevent dehydration, which can lead to complications such as mental confusion or kidney failure.

Monitoring intake allows early detection of signs of undernutrition or dehydration, facilitating rapid intervention.

The caregiver's role in monitoring intake and swallowing disorders

1. **Careful observation of the patient**

   The caregiver must be alert to signs of swallowing difficulties:
   - **Coughing or choking during or after meals**: Indicates a possible false route.
   - **Voice changes**: A hoarse or wet voice may suggest the presence of fluid in the respiratory tract.
   - **Food residues in the mouth**: Indicates incomplete chewing or swallowing.
   - **Refusal to eat or reduced appetite**: May be linked to fear of choking or discomfort when swallowing.
   - **Involuntary weight loss**: A sign of potential malnutrition.

2. **Registration of contributions**
   - **Quantifying meals eaten**: Note the proportion of the plate finished, and the foods refused or preferred.
   - **Fluid intake monitoring**: Record the quantity of beverages consumed daily.

- **Use of monitoring sheets**: Enables traceability and facilitates communication with the care team.

3. **Adapting your diet**

    - **Modified textures**: Offer blended, chopped or thickened foods as recommended.
    - **Food variety**: Offer appetizing meals to stimulate the desire to eat.
    - **Meal frequency**: divide the diet into several small meals to facilitate ingestion.

4. **Assistance with meals**

    - **Patient positioning**: Place the patient in an upright sitting position, head tilted slightly forward to facilitate swallowing.
    - **Suitable pace**: give patients time to chew and swallow, avoid rushing them.
    - **Encouragement and support**: Motivating patients, rewarding their efforts, creating a calm atmosphere.

5. **Collaboration with the multidisciplinary team**

    - **Reporting observations**: Inform the nurse or doctor of any difficulties observed.
    - **Participation in follow-up meetings**: Contribute to the development of the nutritional care plan.
    - **Coordination with speech therapists**: These professionals can suggest swallowing re-education exercises.

Strategies for managing swallowing disorders

1. **Safe feeding techniques**

   - **Food of appropriate consistency**: Use thickened liquids for beverages, avoid dry or sticky foods.
   - **Portion size**: Offer small bites to facilitate chewing and swallowing.
   - **Avoid distractions**: Limit surrounding stimuli so that the patient can concentrate on the act of eating.

2. **Stimulation exercises**

   - **Sensory stimulation**: Use foods with strong flavors to stimulate swallowing reflexes.
   - **Facial massage**: Under the guidance of a professional, perform massages to strengthen the muscles involved.

3. **Patient and family education**

   - **Inform about risks**: Explain the importance of following recommendations to prevent complications.
   - **Involve family and friends**: train them in safe feeding techniques.

Preventing complications related to swallowing disorders

False routes can lead to inhalation pneumonitis, a serious infection of the lungs. To prevent these complications:

- **Postprandial monitoring**: Observe patient after meals for signs of respiratory distress.
- **Rigorous oral hygiene**: Keep your mouth clean to reduce the bacterial load and the risk of infection in the event of a false route.

- **Post-meal positioning**: Keep the patient seated for at least 30 minutes after eating.

Managing undernutrition and dehydration

1. **Early detection**
   - **Regular weighing**: Monitor the patient's weight to detect any significant variations.
   - **Intake assessment**: Compare intake quantities with estimated nutritional requirements.

2. **Nutritional intervention**
   - **Oral nutritional supplements**: On medical prescription, offer calorie- and protein-rich supplements.
   - **Reinforced hydration**: Offer drinks regularly, giving preference to liquids adapted to dysphagia.

3. **Customized approach**
   - **Taking preferences into account**: Adapting menus to the patient's tastes to stimulate appetite.
   - **Psychological support**: Address any emotional factors influencing eating, such as depression or anxiety.

Continuing education and skills development

The caregiver must keep abreast of best practices to improve care:

- **Participate in specific training courses**: workshops on swallowing, nutrition in geriatrics, techniques to assist with feeding.
- **Collaborate with specialists**: Speech therapists, dieticians and occupational therapists can provide additional expertise.
- **Self-assessment**: Reflect on your practices and seek to improve them based on feedback from your team and patients.

Mobilization and Travel

- Safe handling techniques

Patient handling is an essential part of the geriatric caregiver's job. It involves mobilizing, transferring or positioning elderly people in a variety of situations, whether to help them get up, move around or perform care tasks. These tasks, although commonplace, involve significant risks for both caregiver and patient if not carried out correctly. Safe handling techniques are designed to prevent accidents, musculoskeletal injuries and ensure patient comfort and safety. Mastering these techniques is therefore essential for effective and sustainable professional practice.

The importance of safe handling techniques

Statistics show that musculoskeletal disorders (MSDs) account for a significant proportion of occupational illnesses among caregivers. Repetitive movements, awkward postures and the handling of heavy loads are all risk factors. What's more, poor handling can lead to falls or injuries to patients, who are particularly vulnerable in geriatric care. Adopting safe techniques can help you to :

1. **Preserve caregiver health**: Reduce the risk of back pain, joint and muscle injuries.

2. **Ensuring patient safety**: Avoiding falls, trauma or discomfort caused by improper handling.
3. **Improving the quality of care**: A good command of techniques promotes patient well-being and reinforces trust in the care-giver-patient relationship.
4. **Optimize efficiency**: Correct, ergonomic movements make tasks run more smoothly and with less fatigue.

Basic principles of safe handling

1. **Ergonomics and biomechanics**

   - **Back posture**: Keep the back straight and aligned, avoid excessive twisting or bending of the spine.
   - **Using your legs**: Bend your knees and use the strength of your thighs to lift, rather than bending forward.
   - **Feet apart**: Adopt a stable position with feet shoulder-width apart for a better base of support.
   - **Load proximity**: Keep the patient or object close to the body to reduce the lever arm and reduce stress on the back.
   - **Breathing**: Synchronize movements with breathing to optimize effort and reduce tension.

2. **Pre-evaluation**

   - **Situation analysis**: Before any manipulation, assess the patient's condition, ability to participate, potential risks and specific needs.
   - **Planning**: Determine the appropriate technique, the technical aids required and enlist the help of a colleague if necessary.
   - **Communication with the patient**: Explain the procedure, obtain the patient's cooperation and ensure understanding.

3. **Use of technical aids**

    - **Transfer devices**: Wheelchairs, lifts, transfer boards, walking belts.
    - **Positioning equipment**: Cushions, headrests, limb supports.
    - **User training**: Know how to operate equipment, check it regularly and follow safety protocols.

Specific handling techniques

1. **Help getting out of bed**

    - **Preparation**: Adjust bed height to ergonomic position, lower bed rails, ensure floor is clear.
    - **Patient position**: Encourage the patient to turn onto his side, then sit on the edge of the bed, using his arms if possible.
    - **Assistance**: Position yourself facing the patient, feet staggered, knees bent, offer support under the shoulders or use a transfer belt.
    - **Transition**: Help the patient to stand up, coordinating movements and avoiding pulling on arms or clothing.

2. **Transfer from bed to chair**

    - **Positioning the chair**: Place the chair on the patient's strong side, brakes engaged, footrests up.
    - **Pivoting technique**: Involve the patient by guiding him/her to pivot and sit in the chair, using a transfer belt if necessary.
    - **Using a lift**: If the patient is unable to participate, use a lift according to safety procedures.

3. **Mobilization in bed**

    - **Raising**: To raise the patient to the head of the bed, position yourself on either side of the bed with a colleague, using a sliding sheet or undersheet.
    - **Change of position**: Help the patient turn onto his side, bending his knees and guiding his shoulders and hips.
    - **Pressure sore prevention**: Alternate positions every two hours, use supports to relieve pressure points.

4. **Walking aids**

    - **Balance assessment**: Check the patient's stability, use a cane or walker if necessary.
    - **Positioning**: Stand slightly behind and to the side of the patient, ready to support him/her in the event of imbalance.
    - **Encouragement**: Motivate the patient, adapt the pace to his/her abilities, take breaks if necessary.

Risk prevention for caregivers

1. **Continuing education**

    - Take part in regular training courses on handling techniques, new technical aids and safety protocols.
    - Update your knowledge of ergonomics and MSD prevention.

2. **Self-evaluation**

    - Be aware of your own physical limits, avoid excessive loads, ask for help when necessary.

- Be aware of the body's signals: pain, tension, fatigue, and take steps to remedy them.

3. **Healthy living**

    - Maintain good physical condition through regular activity, strengthening back and leg muscles.
    - Eat a balanced diet and get enough rest.

Patient risk prevention

1. **Communication and consent**

    - Keep the patient informed at every stage, and obtain his or her agreement and involvement.
    - Be attentive to reactions and expressions of pain or discomfort.

2. **Environmental safety**

    - Make sure the floor is clear of obstacles or liquids that could cause slipping.
    - Check that equipment is in good condition: brakes working, no defects on devices.

3. **Adapting to the patient's abilities**

    - Take into account the patient's physical, cognitive or sensory limitations.
    - Adapt techniques to your height, weight and strength.

Use of technical aids

Technical aids are invaluable tools for facilitating handling while reducing risks:

1. **Patient lifts**
    - **Types** : Mobile, rail-mounted, vertical lift.
    - **Procedure**: Choose the right harness, check the maximum authorized weight, follow the installation steps in complete safety.
    - **Benefits**: Reduces caregiver physical effort, increases patient comfort and safety.

2. **Transfer boards**
    - **Use**: to enable the patient to slide from one surface to another (bed to chair, chair to toilet).
    - **Technique**: Place the board under the patient, make sure it's well positioned, guide the movement gently.

3. **Transfer belts**
    - **Function**: To provide a secure grip to help the patient stand up or walk.
    - **Precautions**: Position the belt at waist level, checking that it's snug but not tight.

4. **Sheets and undersheets**
    - **Purpose**: to reduce friction during mobilization in bed and make it easier to raise or turn the patient.
    - **Technique**: Place the sliding sheet under the patient, using coordinated movements with a colleague.

Relational approach to handling

1. **Empathy and respect**
    - Treat patients with dignity, respect their privacy and avoid sudden or invasive gestures.

- Take into account fears, pain and reluctance, and respond to them with patience.

2. **Encouragement and enhancement**

    - Praise patients for their efforts, however modest, to boost their confidence and motivation.
    - Involve the patient as much as possible, giving clear, simple instructions.

3. **Active listening**

    - Be attentive to needs expressed verbally or non-verbally.
    - Adapt interventions according to patient feedback.

Regulations and responsibilities

1. **Compliance with corporate protocols**

    - Know and apply the plant's handling procedures.
    - Participate in mandatory training and comply with safety instructions.

2. **Legal liability**

    - In the event of an accident due to improper handling, the caregiver may be held liable.
    - Document incidents, inform line management and contribute to analysis to prevent recurrences.

3. **Professional ethics**

    - Putting patient safety and well-being first, even in the face of time and resource constraints.
    - Refuse to carry out risky maneuvers without the appropriate means.

- Use of technical aids (walkers, wheelchairs)

Technical aids such as walkers and wheelchairs play an essential role in the care of geriatric patients. They promote mobility, autonomy and safety for patients with physical or functional limitations. The caregiver, through his or her knowledge and expertise, is a key player in the appropriate use of these devices, helping to improve patients' quality of life.

The importance of technical aids in geriatrics

As we age, many patients experience a reduction in their motor skills, whether due to chronic illness, neurological disorders or muscular weakness. Technical aids help to compensate for these limitations, providing physical support and preventing falls. They also encourage active participation in daily activities, boosting self-esteem and a sense of independence.

Using walkers

Walkers, also known as *walking frames*, are devices that help people who have difficulty walking or maintaining their balance. They provide stable, secure support, enabling patients to move around with greater confidence.

Types of walkers

1. **Fixed walkers**: Rigid structures without wheels, offering maximum stability. They require the patient to lift them slightly to move forward, which may require greater physical effort.

2. **Rolling walkers**: Equipped with two wheels at the front and runners or wheels at the back. They facilitate movement without having to lift the device.

3. **Rollators** : Four-wheeled walkers, often with brakes, seat and basket. They are suitable for longer journeys and offer the possibility of resting.

Indications for the use of walkers

- **Balance disorders**: Patients at risk of falls due to instability.

- **Muscular weakness**: reduced leg strength due to neurological or muscular pathologies.

- **Post-surgical recovery**: After orthopedic surgery, such as hip or knee replacement.

- **Joint pain**: osteoarthritis or other conditions limiting mobility.

Role of the caregiver in the use of walkers

1. **Assessment and choice of walker**

    - **Adapting the device**: Make sure the walker is adapted to the patient's height, weight and abilities.

    - **Height adjustment**: Handles should be at the height of the patient's hips, allowing slight elbow flexion.

2. *Technical training*

    - **Positioning**: Teach the patient to stand up straight, between the handles, looking straight ahead.

    - **Movement**: Explain how to move the walker forward one step, then walk with alternating legs, in sync with the device.

    - **Using the brakes** (for rollators): Show how to use the brakes to stop or sit down safely.

3. **Safety and fall prevention**

    - **Safe environment**: Check that the floor is clear, with no obstacles or mats to cause tripping.

    - **Supervision**: Accompany the patient during initial trials, be ready to intervene in the event of imbalance.

    - **Appropriate footwear**: Wear non-slip, closed-toe shoes.

4. **Encouragement and support**

    - **Motivation**: Encourage patients to use walkers to maintain their independence.

    - **Patience**: Respect the patient's pace, giving him or her time to adapt to the device.

Wheelchair use

Wheelchairs are essential for patients who cannot walk or whose mobility is severely limited. They enable movement both indoors and outdoors, facilitating access to social and daily activities.

Wheelchair types

1. **Manual wheelchairs**

    - **Standard wheelchairs**: Propelled by the patient (propulsion circles) or pushed by a third party. They are foldable and relatively light.

    - **Transport wheelchairs**: Lighter, with small rear wheels, designed to be pushed by an attendant.

2. **Electric wheelchairs**

    ○ **Motorized**: Joystick-controlled, suitable for patients with limited arm strength or endurance.

    ○ **Advanced features**: some models allow the seat to be tilted, raised or lowered.

Guidelines for wheelchair use

- **Severe paralysis or weakness**: inability to walk due to neurological damage (paraplegia, hemiplegia).

- **Degenerative diseases**: multiple sclerosis, neuromuscular diseases.

- **Limited endurance**: Inability to cover long distances due to cardiac or respiratory problems.

- **Disabling pain**: Severe arthritis or other conditions limiting mobility.

The caregiver's role in wheelchair use

1. **Adaptation and comfort**

    ○ **Chair adjustment**: Ensure that the seat, footrests and armrests are adjusted for patient comfort and postural support.

    ○ **Pressure sore prevention cushions**: Install suitable cushions to prevent prolonged pressure.

2. **User training**

    ○ **Manual propulsion**: Teach the patient how to use the propulsion circles, maneuver and brake.

    ○ **Safety**: Show how to handle the brakes, avoid obstacles and use ramps safely.

3. **Secure transfers**

    - **From bed to chair**: Use appropriate transfer techniques, with or without technical aids (transfer boards, lifts).
    - **Correct positioning**: Ensure that the patient is correctly seated, with feet on footrests and back supported.

4. **Care and maintenance**

    - **Regular checks**: Check the condition of wheels, brakes and structure to ensure proper operation.
    - **Hygiene**: Clean the chair to maintain a healthy environment.

Promoting independence and mobility

The caregiver must encourage the patient to actively participate in his/her movements, according to his/her abilities:

- **Confidence-building**: Valuing patients' progress, reassuring them of their skills.
- **Gradual adaptation**: Introduce technical aids gradually, as the patient's condition evolves.
- **Realistic goals**: Set achievable goals to maintain motivation.

Collaboration with the multidisciplinary team

1. **Physiotherapists and occupational therapists**

    - **Needs assessment**: These professionals can recommend the most appropriate type of technical aid.

- **Rehabilitation programs**: Working together to integrate the use of aids into rehabilitation exercises.

2. **Doctors and nurses**

    - **Medical follow-up**: keep patients informed of their mobility, report any difficulties or complications.
    - **Prescription management**: Ensure that technical aids are prescribed and financed in accordance with current regulations.

Safety and risk prevention

1. **Staff training**

    - **Knowledge of devices** : The caregiver must be trained in the correct use of the various technical aids.
    - **Regular updates**: Participate in ongoing training to keep abreast of new technologies and best practices.

2. **Patient awareness**

    - **Clear instructions**: Provide simple explanations and demonstrate the steps to be taken.
    - **Precautions**: Inform about potential risks, such as tipping over in the wheelchair or slipping with the walker.

3. **Adapting to the environment**

    - **Accessibility**: Make sure spaces are clear, passageways are wide enough and floors are not slippery.
    - **Signage**: Install visual cues to help patients find their way around.

Ethical and relational aspects

1. **Respect for dignity**

    - **Autonomy**: Encouraging patients to use technical aids to maintain their independence.
    - **Patient choice**: Respect preferences and misgivings, discussing benefits and addressing concerns.

2. **Empathetic communication**

    - **Listening**: Taking into account the difficulties or fears expressed by the patient.
    - **Support**: Offer supportive guidance, reward efforts and successes.

- Preventing falls and maintaining independence

Falls among the elderly are a major public health issue. They can have serious consequences for the physical, psychological and social health of seniors, sometimes leading to significant loss of independence. Preventing these falls is therefore essential to encourage homecare, preserve quality of life and reduce healthcare costs. The caregiver plays a key role in this prevention, adopting a comprehensive approach that encompasses risk assessment, the implementation of appropriate measures and support for patient autonomy.

Understanding fall risk factors

Falls are often the result of a combination of intrinsic (person-related) and extrinsic (environment-related) factors:

1. **Intrinsic factors** :

     - **Physical changes**: Muscular weakness, balance problems, impaired vision or hearing, chronic illnesses (such as osteoarthritis, diabetes, cardiovascular disease).
     - **Cognitive disorders**: Dementia, confusion, attention disorders that can affect hazard perception.
     - **Drug side effects**: Some medications may cause dizziness, orthostatic hypotension or drowsiness.
     - **History of falls**: A previous fall increases the risk of future falls.

2. **Extrinsic factors** :

     - **Unsuitable home environment**: slippery floors, inadequate lighting, lack of handrails or grab bars.
     - **Inappropriate footwear**: ill-fitting shoes, slippery soles or high heels.
     - **Objects in the way**: loose carpets, trailing electrical wires, poorly positioned furniture.

Fall prevention strategies

Falls prevention is based on a multidimensional approach, aimed at reducing risk factors and strengthening the patient's abilities:

1. **Customized risk assessment**

    - **Complete medical check-up**: Work with the medical team to identify medical conditions contributing to the risk of falls.
    - **Environmental analysis**: Visit the patient's home to identify potential hazards and suggest accommodations.
    - **Functional assessment**: Test the patient's balance, muscle strength, mobility and cognitive abilities.

2. **Improving the environment**

    - **Adequate lighting**: Install lamps in dark areas, use night lights at night.
    - **Securing floors**: Fix carpets, eliminate obstacles, choose non-slip coverings.
    - **Installation of technical aids**: Grab bars in the bathroom, handrails on stairs, shower seats.
    - **Space organization**: keep frequently-used objects within easy reach to avoid dangerous stretching or climbing.

3. **Promoting physical activity**

    - **Muscle-strengthening exercises**: Encourage regular activities to strengthen leg and trunk muscles.
    - **Balance and coordination activities**: Tai-chi, yoga, specific exercises recommended by a physiotherapist.
    - **Adapting exercises**: Offer activities adapted to the patient's abilities and preferences to ensure regular and safe practice.

4. **Medication management**

    - **Medication review**: Work with the doctor or pharmacist to identify high-risk drugs and adjust prescriptions if necessary.
    - **Side-effect education**: Inform the patient of the symptoms to watch out for and the importance of reporting any adverse effects.

5. **Education and awareness**

    - **Inform the patient**: Explain the risks of falling, the possible consequences and the importance of preventive measures.
    - **Involve the family**: Make family members aware of the risks and the adjustments needed to support the patient.
    - **Safe movement techniques**: Teach patients how to stand up properly, use walking aids and avoid sudden movements.

6. **Use of technical aids**

    - **Mobility aids**: canes, walkers, wheelchairs adapted to the patient's needs.
    - **User training**: to ensure that the patient masters the operation of these aids for safe and effective use.
    - **Regular maintenance**: Check the condition of devices to prevent mechanical failure.

Maintaining patient autonomy

Preventing falls does not mean restricting patients' activities, but rather adapting them to preserve their independence:

1. **Encouraging independence**

- **Active participation**: Involving patients in decisions concerning their environment and routines.
- **Adapting activities**: proposing safe alternatives for everyday tasks, using ergonomic tools or simplified techniques.
- **Valuing abilities**: Emphasize the patient's achievements to boost self-confidence.

2. **Emotional support**

   - **Empathetic listening**: Recognize fears related to falls, such as the fear of dependence or loss of autonomy.
   - **Stress management**: Offer relaxation techniques, encourage participation in social activities to reduce anxiety.

3. **Personalized care planning**

   - **Realistic goals**: Establish goals with the patient that are adapted to his or her abilities and wishes.
   - **Regular follow-up**: Periodically reassess the patient's needs and adjust interventions accordingly.

The caregiver's role in preventing falls and maintaining autonomy

The caregiver is on the front line in implementing prevention strategies and supporting the patient's autonomy:

1. **Careful observation**

   - **Detecting changes** : Monitor changes in the patient's physical or mental state that may increase the risk of falling.

- ◦ **Reporting**: Communicate quickly with the care team if a problem is identified.

2. **Daily support**

    - ◦ **Safe assistance**: Help the patient move around using safe handling techniques.
    - ◦ **Stimulation of activity**: Encourage patients to participate in daily activities, respecting their pace.

3. **Education and advice**

    - ◦ **Sharing information**: Explain preventive measures clearly and in a way that is adapted to the patient's level of understanding.
    - ◦ **Practical demonstration**: Show how to use technical aids or perform movements safely.

4. **Collaboration with the multidisciplinary team**

    - ◦ **Teamwork**: Participate in coordination meetings, share observations and suggestions.
    - ◦ **Ongoing training**: Keeping up to date with best practices and new recommendations in falls prevention.

Urinary and faecal elimination

- Assistance with natural needs

Assisting with natural needs is a fundamental component of the caregiver's role in geriatrics. It encompasses assisting the elderly with their elimination functions, i.e. with urination and defecation, while ensuring that their dignity, comfort and privacy are preserved. This support is essential to maintain patients' quality of life, prevent medical complications linked to incontinence or constipation, and promote their psychological well-being.

Understanding the natural needs of the elderly

With age, many factors can affect elimination functions:

- **Physiological changes**: Decreased muscle tone, reduced bladder or bowel sensitivity, and hormonal changes can influence micturition and defecation.
- **Associated pathologies**: Diseases such as Alzheimer's, diabetes, stroke or Parkinson's can lead to urinary or bowel problems.
- **Drug side effects**: Some drugs may cause constipation, diarrhea or increased urinary frequency.
- **Psychological factors**: Depression, anxiety or stress can affect elimination habits.

The caregiver's role in assisting with natural needs

1. **Preserving dignity and respect**

    - **Privacy**: Always ensure that the patient is protected from prying eyes when attending to natural needs. Close doors, use screens if necessary.
    - **Caring communication**: Approach the subject tactfully, avoid pejorative language, and respect the patient's feelings.
    - **Consent**: Ask permission before intervening, even if the patient is used to receiving help.

2. **Assistance tailored to individual needs**

    - **Ability assessment**: Determine whether the patient can go to the toilet alone, with partial or total assistance.

- **Use of appropriate equipment**: bedpans, commode chairs, urinals, absorbent pads, depending on specific needs.
- **Mobilization assistance**: Facilitate patient movement to the toilet using safe handling techniques.

3. **Preventing complications**

   - **Elimination monitoring**: Observe the frequency, quantity, color and consistency of urine and stools, and report any abnormalities to the care team.
   - **Prevent urinary tract infections**: Encourage good personal hygiene and ensure adequate hydration.
   - **Prevent constipation**: Eat a high-fiber diet and encourage appropriate physical activity.

4. **Promoting autonomy**

   - **Encouragement**: Motivate patients to take an active part in elimination care to the best of their ability.
   - **Adapting the environment**: Install grab bars, raise toilets, use devices to facilitate access to washrooms.
   - **Scheduling**: Establish routines for going to the toilet at regular times, respecting the patient's habits.

5. **Incontinence management**

   - **Personalized approach**: Assess the causes of incontinence and adapt interventions accordingly.

- **Choice of pads**: Select absorbent pads adapted to the degree of incontinence, and ensure regular changes for the patient's comfort.
- **Psychological support**: understanding the emotional impact of incontinence, offering empathetic support, avoiding stigmatization.

Specific assistance techniques

1. **Help with urination**

    - **Positioning**: Facilitate a comfortable position for the patient, either sitting or standing, depending on his/her abilities.
    - **Reflex stimulation**: Use techniques to facilitate urination, such as the sound of running water or applying a warm compress to the lower abdomen.
    - **Adapted urinals**: For men, offer portable urinals if moving around is difficult.

2. **Defecation aid**

    - **Comfort**: Ensure a physiological position, with feet firmly planted, possibly raised to encourage the evacuation reflex.
    - **Sufficient time**: Let the patient take the necessary time, without rushing, to avoid stress that can inhibit defecation.
    - **Abdominal massage**: In case of constipation, massage gently in the direction of transit to stimulate intestinal activity.

Hygiene and infection control

- **Hand hygiene**: Wash hands before and after use, use single-use gloves to prevent transmission of germs.

- **Intimate hygiene care**: Gently cleanse intimate areas after elimination, respecting the direction of cleansing (from front to back in women) to avoid infection.
- **Waste management**: Dispose of soiled protection in accordance with protocols, ensuring environmentally safe disposal.

Communication and interpersonal skills

- **Active listening**: Listening to the patient's concerns, both verbal and non-verbal.
- **Empathy**: Acknowledging the patient's feelings of shame or embarrassment, reassuring them that these needs are normal.
- **Information**: Explain procedures, answer questions, involve patients in decisions concerning their care plan.

Collaboration with the care team

- **Reporting abnormalities**: Inform the nurse or doctor of any symptoms such as painful urination, blood in the urine, persistent diarrhoea or prolonged constipation.
- **Participation in follow-up meetings**: Contribute to the development and adaptation of the care plan by sharing relevant observations.
- **Ongoing training**: Keep abreast of new practices, innovative techniques and institutional protocols concerning assistance with natural needs.

Ethical approach and respect for patient rights

- **Confidentiality**: Respecting professional secrecy, not divulging personal information without the patient's consent.
- **Informed consent**: Ensuring that the patient understands and accepts the proposed interventions.
- **Non-judgmental**: Adopt a neutral attitude, without criticism or mockery, whatever the situation.

Managing special situations

1. Patients with cognitive disorders

- **Adapted approach**: Use simple sentences and gestures to facilitate understanding.
- **Routines**: Maintain a regular schedule to create reference points.
- **Increased monitoring**: Be alert to non-verbal signs indicating the need to eliminate.

2. Restless or resistant patients

- **Calm and patient**: Avoid confrontation, use distraction techniques.
- **Safety**: Ensuring a safe environment, preventing the risk of falls.

- Incontinence management

Incontinence management is an essential aspect of geriatric care for the elderly. Incontinence, whether urinary or faecal, affects a significant proportion of the senior population and can have a major impact on patients' quality of life, dignity and psychological well-being. The caregiver plays a central role in the recognition, management and support of people suffering from incontinence, working closely with the multidisciplinary team to provide appropriate and respectful care.

Understanding incontinence

Incontinence is defined as the involuntary loss of urine or faeces, resulting from a malfunction of the urinary or digestive system. In the elderly, several factors can contribute to the onset of incontinence:

1. **Age-related physiological changes**: Aging leads to reduced pelvic floor muscle elasticity, reduced bladder capacity and impaired sphincter control.

2. **Associated pathologies**: Conditions such as Parkinson's disease, stroke, dementia, diabetes or multiple sclerosis can affect sphincter control.

3. **Drug side effects**: Some treatments, such as diuretics, sedatives or anticholinergics, can influence urinary frequency or the ability to retain urine.

4. **Environmental and psychological factors**: Physical barriers, reduced mobility, confusion or depression can hinder access to the toilet or recognition of the need to eliminate.

Impact of incontinence on the patient

Incontinence has many consequences:

- **Physical**: Increased risk of urinary tract infections, skin irritation and bedsores.
- **Psychological**: Feelings of shame, embarrassment and anxiety, leading to social isolation or depression.
- **Social**: reduced participation in activities, withdrawal, stigmatization.

The caregiver's role in incontinence management

1. **Assessment and observation**

    - **Careful monitoring**: record frequency, volume and circumstances of incontinence episodes.
    - **Identify associated signs**: Pain, burning, blood in urine, unusual odor.
    - **Communication with the patient**: Approach the subject tactfully to gather information about feelings and habits.

2. **Setting up a personalized care plan**

    - **Collaborate with the care team**: Participate in the development of a care plan adapted to the patient's specific needs.
    - **Behavioural techniques**: Encourage the patient to follow a program of programmed micturition, and practice pelvic floor strengthening exercises (Kegel exercises) under medical supervision.
    - **Adapting the environment**: Facilitate access to toilets by eliminating obstacles, installing grab bars and ensuring that toilets are well-lit and signposted.

3. **Use of appropriate protection and devices**

    - **Selecting pads**: Choose absorbent pads adapted to the degree of incontinence, taking into account comfort and discretion for the patient.
    - **Device management** : Ensure regular changes of protection to maintain hygiene and prevent skin irritation.
    - **Training in use**: Explain to the patient how to use the protectors, if his or her condition allows, to promote autonomy.

4. **Hygiene care and prevention of complications**

    - **Rigorous skin hygiene**: gently cleanse the skin after each incontinence episode with mild products, and dry carefully to avoid maceration.
    - **Application of barrier creams**: Use protective ointments to prevent irritation and dermatitis associated with incontinence.
    - **Monitoring for signs of infection**: Be alert to any redness, pain or suspicious odours, and inform the nurse or doctor if necessary.

5. Psychological support and preservation of dignity

- **Empathic approach**: Acknowledge the patient's emotions, reassure him or her that incontinence is common and that there's no need to feel guilty.
- **Respect for privacy**: Ensuring that care is provided discreetly, preserving the patient's modesty.
- **Encouragement**: Valuing the patient's efforts, motivating them to participate in social activities and maintain a positive self-image.

Collaboration with the multidisciplinary team

- **Nurses and doctors**: Pass on observations, participate in adjustments to medication or suggest additional tests.
- **Physiotherapists**: Working together to set up perineal rehabilitation programs.
- **Occupational therapists**: Adapting the patient's environment, proposing technical aids to facilitate access to bathroom facilities.
- **Psychologists**: Refer patients if signs of emotional distress or depression are detected.

Patient and family education

1. Clear, appropriate information

- **Explaining the causes**: Helping patients and their families understand the mechanisms of incontinence.
- **Presentation of options**: explain the different management strategies and the advantages and disadvantages of each approach.

2. **Practical advice**

    - **Eating habits**: ensure adequate hydration, avoid bladder irritants such as caffeine, alcohol or spicy foods.
    - **Clothing habits**: Wear clothes that are easy to remove for quick access to the toilet.
    - **Situation management** : Plan outings taking into account needs (location of public toilets, carrying spare protection).

3. **Involving family and friends**

    - **Emotional support**: Encourage the family to adopt an understanding, non-judgmental attitude.
    - **Participating in care**: training caregivers in assistance techniques, while respecting the patient's limits.

Incontinence prevention

- **Regular physical activity**: Encourage exercises that strengthen pelvic muscles and improve overall mobility.
- **Medical surveillance**: Encourage regular check-ups to detect conditions that may cause incontinence.
- **Medication management** : Work with physician to adjust treatments that may influence bladder or bowel function.

Ethical approach and respect for patient rights

- **Autonomy**: Respect the patient's choice of incontinence management methods.
- **Confidentiality**: Protect personal information, share medical data only with the professionals concerned.
- **Informed consent**: Ensuring that the patient understands the proposed interventions and consents to them freely.

- Diuresis and stool monitoring

Monitoring diuresis and stool output is an essential component of care for the elderly in geriatric medicine. It enables the monitoring of hydration, renal and digestive function, as well as the early detection of possible imbalances or pathologies. The caregiver plays a key role in this monitoring, carefully observing intake and elimination, recording data and communicating effectively with the nursing team. This approach helps to ensure comprehensive, preventive care tailored to the specific needs of elderly patients.

Importance of diuresis and stool monitoring

As people age, their renal and digestive functions undergo physiological changes that can affect their water, electrolyte and nutritional balance. Decreased glomerular filtration, reduced sensation of thirst and impaired intestinal motility are all factors likely to lead to complications such as dehydration, renal failure, constipation or diarrhea.

Regular monitoring of diuresis (the amount of urine excreted) and stool enables :

- Assess the patient's hydration status.
- Detect early signs of renal failure or urinary tract infection.
- Monitor the effectiveness of diuretic or hydric treatments.
- Identify digestive disorders such as constipation, diarrhea or gastrointestinal bleeding.
- Adjust nutritional and water intake according to needs.

Role of the caregiver in surveillance

The caregiver, by virtue of his or her proximity to the patient, is in the front line for observing and gathering the necessary information:

1. **Data collection**

    ○ **Diuresis quantification**: Measure the quantity of urine eliminated over a given period (usually 24 hours), using suitable devices such as graduated urinals, urine bags or commode chairs.
    ○ **Observation of urinary characteristics**: Note color, transparency, odor, presence of sediment or blood (hematuria).
    ○ **Stool recording**: Record stool frequency, consistency (according to the Bristol scale), color, odor, and the presence of abnormal signs such as blood (melena or rectorrhagia), mucus or parasites.

2. **Documentation**

    ○ **Monitoring sheets**: Fill in the water input and output monitoring sheets accurately, indicating times, quantities and relevant observations.
    ○ **Traceability**: Ensure legible writing, use appropriate units of measurement (milliliters for liquids), and comply with plant protocols.

3. **Communication with the care team**

    ○ **Reporting abnormalities**: Promptly inform the nurse or doctor in the event of significant changes or alarming signs (anuria, oliguria, polyuria, acute diarrhea, prolonged constipation).
    ○ **Participate in communications**: Sharing information during changeovers, helping to draw up the care plan by providing concrete information.

Monitoring techniques

1. **Diuresis measurement**

    - **Urine collection**: Use clean, appropriate devices, make sure the patient understands the need to collect all micturition, assist if necessary.
    - **Hygiene precautions**: Wear single-use gloves, wash hands before and after use, clean and disinfect equipment after use.
    - **Quantification**: Measure urine volume using a graduated container, noting quantities at each micturition or over defined time intervals.

2. **Stool monitoring**

    - **Direct observation**: When changing or helping with the toilet, discreetly observe stool characteristics.
    - **Bristol scale**: Use this scale to classify stool consistency from type 1 (very hard) to type 7 (liquid).
    - **Collection if necessary**: If further tests are required, collect a stool sample in accordance with protocols.

3. **Tracking entries and exits**

    - **Water balance**: Compare water intake (drinks, infusions) with losses (urine, stools, vomit, perspiration) to assess the patient's water balance.
    - **Adapting care**: Based on results, contribute to adjusting intake in collaboration with the care team.

Signs to watch out for and action to take

1. **Urinary anomalies**

   - **Anuria**: Total absence of urine for more than 12 hours, medical emergency.
   - **Oliguria**: Diuresis of less than 500 ml per 24 hours, which may indicate dehydration or renal failure.
   - **Polyuria**: Diuresis of more than 2.5 liters per 24 hours, which may be linked to diabetes insipidus or diabetes mellitus.
   - **Hematuria**: Presence of blood in the urine, requiring medical investigation.

2. **Stool abnormalities**

   - **Constipation**: Absence of stools for more than three days, or hard stools that are difficult to evacuate.
   - **Diarrhea**: frequent liquid stools, risk of dehydration and electrolyte imbalance.
   - **Blood in stools**: presence of red (rectorrhagia) or black (melena) blood, a potential sign of digestive hemorrhage.
   - **Abdominal pain**: associated with transit disorders, may indicate occlusion or infection.

Relational and ethical approach

- **Respect for dignity**: Approach the subject with tact, respect the patient's privacy, ensure the confidentiality of information gathered.
- **Appropriate communication**: Explain the importance of monitoring, reassure patients and answer their questions sympathetically.

- **Empathy**: Understand any discomfort or discomfort related to these observations, adopt a professional and understanding attitude.

Interprofessional collaboration

- **Teamwork**: Working closely with nurses, doctors and dieticians to provide comprehensive care.
- **Ongoing training**: Participate in training sessions on monitoring techniques, hygiene protocols, clinical signs to recognize.
- **Participation in meetings**: Contribute to discussions on the patient's condition, share observations to adjust the care plan.

Prevention and education

- **Adequate hydration**: Encourage patients to drink regularly, adapting intake according to needs and medical restrictions.
- **Balanced diet**: Eat a high-fiber diet to prevent constipation, and adapt diets in case of diarrhea.
- **Physical activity**: Stimulate patient mobility, even in moderation, to promote intestinal transit.

Rest and Sleep

- The importance of sleep-wake rhythms

The sleep-wake rhythm, also known as the circadian cycle, is a fundamental biological process that regulates periods of wakefulness and sleep over a 24-hour period. In the elderly, this rhythm can be significantly altered by physiological, environmental and pathological factors. Understanding the importance of this rhythm and its impact on seniors' health is essential for geriatric professionals, including caregivers, who play a key role in promoting the well-being and quality of life of the elderly.

Understanding the sleep-wake rhythm

The circadian rhythm is orchestrated by a biological clock located in the hypothalamus, more precisely in the suprachiasmatic nucleus. This internal clock synchronizes bodily functions with day-night cycles, influencing body temperature, hormone secretion, appetite and sleep. Melatonin, a hormone produced by the pineal gland, plays a crucial role in inducing sleep by signalling to the body that it's time to rest.

Alterations in sleep-wake rhythms in the elderly

As we age, several changes can disrupt our sleep-wake rhythm:

1. **Decreased melatonin production**: Melatonin secretion tends to decline with age, which can lead to difficulties in initiating and maintaining sleep.

2. **Changes in sleep structure**: the elderly spend less time in deep sleep (stage N3) and REM sleep, crucial phases for physical and cognitive recovery. Sleep becomes lighter and more fragmented.

3. **Sleep phase advancement**: Seniors often tend to go to bed earlier in the evening and wake up earlier in the morning, which may not correspond to their social or family environment.

4. **Increased sensitivity to environmental factors**: noise, light or comfort conditions can have a greater impact on sleep in the elderly.

5. **Presence of pathologies**: Chronic illnesses such as sleep apnea, restless legs syndrome, chronic pain or

cognitive disorders such as dementia can affect sleep quality and quantity.

6. **Polypharmacy**: Taking multiple medications can have sleep-disrupting side effects, such as insomnia or daytime sleepiness.

Consequences of sleep-wake rhythm disorders

Disturbances in the sleep-wake cycle can have a significant impact on the health and well-being of the elderly:

1. **Impaired cognitive functions**: Insufficient or poor-quality sleep can lead to problems with memory, attention and concentration, increasing the risk of confusion or dementia.

2. **Increased risk of falls**: Daytime drowsiness or frequent nocturnal awakenings can cause dizziness or imbalance, increasing the risk of falls and injuries.

3. **Weakened immune system**: Disturbed sleep can reduce the body's ability to fight infection and recover from illness.

4. **Impact on mental health**: Sleep disorders are associated with an increased risk of depression, anxiety and irritability.

5. **Exacerbation of chronic diseases**: Conditions such as hypertension, diabetes or heart disease can be aggravated by insufficient sleep.

The role of the caregiver in promoting a healthy sleep-wake rhythm

The caregiver can implement various strategies to help the elderly maintain a balanced sleep-wake rhythm:

1. **Assessment and observation**

    - **Monitoring sleep habits**: Record bedtime and wake-up times, sleep duration, nocturnal awakenings, daytime naps.

    - **Identifying disruptive factors**: Observe factors that may interfere with sleep, such as noise, light, pain or frequent urination.

    - **Communication with the care team**: Transmit observations to nurses and doctors to adjust care plan if necessary.

2. **Improved sleeping environment**

    - **Bed comfort**: Ensure that mattresses, pillows and bed linen are suitable and comfortable.

    - **Light control**: Use blackout curtains to reduce outside light, and sleep masks if appropriate.

    - **Noise reduction**: Limit noise sources, use earplugs or devices emitting soothing sounds.

    - **Room temperature**: Maintain a pleasant temperature in the room, neither too hot nor too cold.

3. **Establishing regular routines**

    - **Fixed schedules**: Encourage the patient to go to bed and get up at regular times to synchronize the biological clock.

    - **Soothing rituals**: Suggest relaxing activities before bedtime, such as reading, listening to soft music or meditating.

- **Limiting naps**: Regulate the duration and frequency of daytime naps to avoid disrupting night-time sleep.

4. **Promoting physical activity and exposure to natural light**
   - **Regular exercise**: Encourage adapted physical activities, such as walking, gardening or gentle gymnastics, to promote natural fatigue.
   - **Daylight**: expose the patient to natural light in the morning to reinforce the circadian rhythm.

5. **Management of medical and drug-related factors**
   - **Pain management**: Collaborate with the care team to effectively manage pain that can disrupt sleep.
   - **Medication evaluation**: Monitor medication side effects, inform doctor if excessive sleepiness or insomnia occurs.
   - **Treatment of specific disorders**: Help set up therapies for sleep disorders such as obstructive sleep apnea.

6. **Education and support**
   - **Patient information**: Explain the importance of good sleep, the consequences of sleep disorders and how to remedy them.
   - **Family involvement**: Make family members aware of the patient's needs, encourage a family environment conducive to sleep.

- **Psychological support**: listening to patients' concerns, offering support in the event of anxiety or depression.

Non-pharmacological approaches to improving sleep

It is often preferable to use non-drug interventions to treat sleep disorders in the elderly:

1. **Relaxation techniques**

    - **Deep breathing**: Teaching breathing exercises to reduce stress and promote sleep.
    - **Progressive muscle relaxation**: Help the patient to gradually relax each muscle group.
    - **Meditation and mindfulness**: offer guided sessions to calm the mind.

2. **Cognitive and behavioral therapy**

    - **Managing negative thoughts**: helping patients to identify and modify anxiety-provoking sleep-related thoughts.
    - **Restricting time spent in bed**: Avoid staying in bed in the event of prolonged insomnia, favoring quiet activities until drowsiness sets in.

3. **Adapting your diet**

    - **Avoid stimulants**: Reduce consumption of caffeine, nicotine and alcohol, especially at the end of the day.
    - **Light evening meals**: Choose easily digestible foods to avoid gastric discomfort.

- **Balanced hydration**: Limit fluid intake in the evening to reduce night-time awakening due to urinary needs.

Precautions concerning sleeping pills

The use of hypnotic drugs should be considered with caution in the elderly, due to the risk of side effects such as confusion, falls or drug interactions. The caregiver must be alert to signs of adverse effects and inform the medical team.

Impact of sleep-wake rhythm on overall health

Maintaining a regular, high-quality sleep-wake rhythm has beneficial effects on :

- **Cognitive function**: Improved memory, attention and reasoning skills.

- **Mood**: Reduced depressive symptoms, irritability and anxiety.

- **Physical health**: boosting the immune system, regulating metabolism, reducing the risk of cardiovascular disease.

- **Quality of life**: Increased energy, better participation in social activities, general sense of well-being.

- Creating a restful environment

Rest is an essential component of well-being and health, particularly for the elderly. A suitable environment can greatly influence the quality of sleep and rest, contributing to physical, mental and emotional recovery. In the context of geriatrics, the design of living spaces to promote rest is of crucial importance. The aim is not only to create an environment conducive to sleep, but also to support the elderly's sense of security, comfort and dignity. The caregiver plays a key role in this process, ensuring that the environment is adapted to the specific needs of each individual.

The importance of a restful environment

With age, sleep undergoes changes: it becomes lighter, less deep, and night-time awakenings are more frequent. In addition, the elderly may be affected by a variety of medical or psychological conditions that disrupt their rest. An unsuitable environment can exacerbate these difficulties, leading to fatigue, irritability, confusion or aggravation of certain pathologies. Conversely, a well-designed space can improve sleep quality, promote relaxation and contribute to better overall health.

Key principles for environmental design

1. **Physical comfort**

    - **Appropriate bedding**: A good quality mattress, neither too firm nor too soft, is essential to support the body and prevent pain. Pillows should be comfortable and offer adequate support for the head and neck.

    - **Temperature control**: The bedroom should be kept at a comfortable temperature, generally between 18 and 20 degrees Celsius. Too high or too low a temperature can disrupt sleep.

    - **Appropriate sleepwear**: Comfortable pyjamas in natural materials like cotton help regulate body temperature and ensure optimum comfort.

2. **Light management**

    - **Darkness at night**: A dark room promotes the production of melatonin, the sleep hormone.

Blackout curtains or shutters can help block out outside light.

- **Soft lighting**: If required, nightlights with adjustable intensity can be installed to enable safe movement without disturbing sleep.

- **Exposure to natural light**: During the day, exposure to daylight helps regulate the circadian rhythm, making it easier to fall asleep in the evening.

3. **Noise reduction**

    - **Soundproofing**: If possible, use sound-absorbing materials to reduce ambient noise. Carpets, thick curtains and acoustic panels can contribute to a quieter atmosphere.

    - **Limiting noise sources**: Avoid noisy activities near the bedroom during sleeping hours. Electronic devices such as television and radio should be used in moderation.

    - **Use soothing sounds**: White noise or relaxing music can help mask disruptive noises and promote relaxation.

4. **Space organization**

    - **Safe layout**: The layout of the room must allow for easy, obstacle-free circulation to prevent falls. Furniture must be arranged in a functional and safe manner.

    - **Personalization**: Incorporating personal objects, photos or familiar decorations can create a sense of comfort and security.

- **Proper storage**: An orderly space reduces stress and facilitates access to necessary items, thus avoiding frustration or nocturnal agitation.

5. **Air quality**
   - **Ventilation**: Good room ventilation is essential for optimum air quality. Opening windows regularly, conditions permitting, can refresh the atmosphere.
   - **Humidity control**: Humidity levels that are too high or too low can affect respiratory comfort. Humidifiers or dehumidifiers can be used to maintain an adequate level.
   - **Avoid irritants**: Limit the use of chemicals or strong perfumes that could cause allergies or irritation.

6. **Promoting soothing rituals**
   - **Bedtime routine**: Encourage relaxing activities before sleep, such as reading, listening to soft music or breathing exercises.
   - **Avoid stimulants**: Reduce consumption of caffeine, nicotine or alcohol at the end of the day, which can disrupt sleep.
   - **Regular schedules**: Maintain constant bedtimes and wake-up times to regulate the biological clock.

The caregiver's role in designing the environment

The caregiver, in collaboration with the nursing team and the family, can intervene in various ways:

- **Needs assessment**: Observe the patient's sleep habits, identify disruptive factors and collect their preferences.

- **Setting up the facilities**: Adapt bedding, organize space, install devices to improve comfort and safety.

- **Communication**: Inform the patient of the changes made, ensure his/her agreement and satisfaction. Explain the importance of certain adjustments for the patient's well-being.

- **Monitoring**: Continue to observe the effectiveness of the accommodations, adjusting if necessary based on patient feedback and clinical observations.

- **Education and advice**: educate patients and their families about best practices for rest, and suggest strategies for managing sleep disorders.

Collaboration with the multidisciplinary team

- **Healthcare professionals**: Work with nurses, doctors and psychologists to identify the medical causes of sleep disorders and implement appropriate interventions.

- **Occupational therapists**: Call on their expertise to optimize the layout of the space, and choose suitable, ergonomic equipment.

- **Physiotherapists**: Integrate adapted physical exercises to promote natural fatigue and improve sleep quality.

Respect for patient preferences and autonomy

It is essential to respect the patient's wishes in terms of environment and routines. The caregiver must take care to:

- **Personalize interventions**: Adapt facilities to the patient's tastes, cultural habits and specific needs.

- **Encourage autonomy**: Encourage patients to participate in the organization of their space, express their preferences and maintain their personal rituals.

- **Avoid infantilization**: Treat patients with respect, avoid making decisions on their behalf without consultation.

Managing special situations

- **Cognitive disorders**: For patients suffering from dementia or confusion, the environment needs to be secure yet soothing. Visual cues, appropriate lighting and familiar objects can help reduce anxiety.

- **Chronic pain**: working with the medical team to manage pain effectively, using adapted sleeping positions and support devices.

- **Anxiety and depression**: Offer relaxation techniques, create a reassuring environment, and encourage dialogue to express concerns.

- Detection of sleep disorders

Sleep is a vital function essential to physical, mental and emotional health. In the elderly, sleep can be disrupted by a variety of factors, leading to disorders that significantly affect their quality of life. Early detection of these disorders is crucial to prevent complications and improve patient well-being. The caregiver, by virtue of his or her proximity to the elderly, plays a decisive role in identifying signs suggestive of sleep disorders. By adopting an attentive, empathetic approach, they make an active contribution to appropriate, effective care.

The importance of sleep in the elderly

With age, sleep undergoes natural changes: it becomes lighter, less deep, and REM sleep phases diminish. These physiological changes can make the elderly more vulnerable to sleep disturbances. Yet quality sleep is essential for :

- **Maintain cognitive functions**: memory consolidation and learning are closely linked to deep sleep phases.
- **Support the immune system**: sufficient rest strengthens the body's ability to fight infection.
- **Preserve emotional balance**: lack of sleep can exacerbate depressive or anxiety symptoms.
- **Ensure proper physical recovery**: sleep enables tissue regeneration and cellular repair.

Main sleep disorders in the elderly

1. **Insomnia**: difficulty falling asleep, frequent awakenings during the night, early awakening in the morning. It can be chronic or transitory, linked to psychological, environmental or medical factors.

2. **Obstructive sleep apnea**: repeated breathing interruptions during sleep due to upper airway obstruction, leading to micro-awakenings and daytime drowsiness.

3. **Restless legs syndrome**: unpleasant sensations in the legs, prompting movement, especially at rest or at night, disrupting sleep.

4. **Circadian rhythm disorders**: desynchronization between the internal sleep-wake rhythm and the external environment, leading to daytime sleepiness or nocturnal insomnia.

5. **Parasomnias**: abnormal sleep behaviors such as sleepwalking, night terrors or nightmares.

Signs suggestive of sleep disorders

The caregiver must be attentive to the following manifestations:

- **Patient complaints**: difficulty falling asleep, persistent fatigue, unrefreshing sleep.
- **Daytime sleepiness**: involuntary falling asleep during the day, difficulty staying awake during quiet activities.
- **Irritability or mood swings**: nervousness, depression, anxiety may result from lack of sleep.
- **Cognitive disorders**: confusion, memory impairment, difficulty concentrating.
- **Unusual behaviours**: nocturnal agitation, incoherent speech during sleep, sleepwalking episodes.
- **Physical signs**: dark circles, reddened eyes, reduced appetite.

The caregiver's role in detecting sleep disorders

1. Careful observation
   The caregiver, present with the patient on a daily basis, is ideally placed to observe the subtle signs of sleep disorders:
   - **Night-time monitoring**: note frequent awakenings, periods of agitation, intense snoring or pauses in breathing.
   - **Daytime observation**: notice drowsiness, sudden onset of sleep, loss of energy.

2. Listening and communication
   - **Open dialogue**: encourage patients to talk about their sleep and their feelings, without minimizing their concerns.

- **Targeted questioning**: ask about sleep habits, bedtime rituals and any nightmares.

3. **Recording information**

    - **Keep a sleep diary**: record bedtimes and wake-up times, night-time awakenings, naps, symptoms observed.
    - **Transmission to the care team**: share observations with nurses and doctors for in-depth assessment.

4. **Identifying contributing factors**

    - **Environment**: check whether noise, light and room temperature can disrupt sleep.
    - **Medication**: be aware that some treatments can affect sleep (stimulants, diuretics, corticoids).
    - **Pain or physical discomfort**: look for signs of unexpressed pain that may interfere with falling asleep.

Strategies for detecting sleep disorders

1. **Training and awareness-raising**

    - **Acquire knowledge**: learn about the different sleep disorders, their signs and consequences.
    - **Staying informed**: keeping up to date with the latest protocols and best practices in geriatric sleep.

2. **Individualized approach**

    - **Get to know the patient**: understand his or her habits, medical history and preferences.

- **Adapting interventions**: proposing personalized solutions to improve sleep (soothing routines, adapted environment).

3. **Interdisciplinary collaboration**
    - **Teamwork**: exchanging information with other professionals (doctors, nurses, psychologists, physiotherapists) to ensure comprehensive care.
    - **Refer to specialists**: if severe disorders are suspected, suggest an assessment by a sleep doctor or neurologist.

The importance of early detection

Identifying sleep disorders early on allows you to :

- **Prevent complications**: drowsiness-related falls, aggravation of chronic illnesses, cognitive disorders.
- **Improving quality of life**: restful sleep contributes to a better mood, greater vitality and increased participation in activities.
- **Adapt treatments**: adjust medications, suggest non-pharmacological therapies (relaxation, light therapy).
- **Support the patient**: help them understand their difficulties, reduce their anxiety, reinforce their sense of control.

Practical tips for caregivers

- **Create an environment conducive to sleep**: make sure the bedroom is quiet, dark and at a pleasant temperature.
- **Encourage healthy sleep habits**: keep regular hours, avoid stimulants at the end of the day, limit prolonged naps.
- **Promote relaxing activities**: gentle exercises, reading, soothing music before bedtime.

- **Avoid night-time disturbances**: minimize night-time interventions, use bedside lamps rather than main lighting.

Ethical and respectful approach

- **Confidentiality**: respect the patient's privacy, do not divulge their difficulties without their consent.
- **Empathy**: show understanding, avoid minimizing complaints or passing judgment.
- **Autonomy**: involving patients in decisions concerning their sleep, respecting their choices and preferences.

Chapter 4

Management of common pathologies

Neurodegenerative diseases

- Alzheimer's disease: signs and support

Alzheimer's disease is a progressive neurodegenerative disorder affecting millions of people worldwide. It is characterized by a progressive deterioration of cognitive functions, leading to memory loss, language, thought and behavior disorders. Understanding the warning signs and knowing how to accompany a person suffering from dementia is essential to providing appropriate support and preserving quality of life. The aim of this book is to shed light on the manifestations of Alzheimer's disease and to suggest approaches for effective, humane support.

Understanding Alzheimer's disease

Alzheimer's disease is the most common form of dementia in the elderly. It results from an abnormal accumulation of proteins in the brain, forming amyloid plaques and neurofibrillary tangles. These abnormalities lead to the degeneration of neurons and reduced transmission of nerve signals. The exact causes remain unknown, but genetic, environmental and lifestyle factors are involved.

Signs and symptoms of Alzheimer's disease

The symptoms of Alzheimer's disease appear progressively and worsen over time. They can be classified into different phases, although the progression varies from person to person.

1. **Early signs**

    - **Recent memory loss**: Difficulty recalling recent events, retaining new information, frequent forgetfulness.
    - **Difficulty planning or solving problems**: inability to follow a recipe, manage invoices, confusion with dates or seasons.

- **Problems with spatial and temporal orientation**: getting lost in familiar places, not knowing what day it is.
- **Language disorders**: difficulty finding the right words, repetition of the same sentences, stopping in the middle of a conversation.
- **Impaired judgment**: Inappropriate decision-making, neglect of personal hygiene, vulnerability to scams.

2. Intermediate phase

    - **Worsening memory problems**: forgetting important events, failing to recognize loved ones, increased disorientation.
    - **Behavioral changes**: Agitation, aggressiveness, depression, anxiety, hallucinations.
    - **Loss of autonomy**: Difficulty performing daily activities (dressing, eating, bathing).
    - **Sleep disorders**: Reversal of sleep-wake rhythm, insomnia, daytime sleepiness.

3. Advanced phase

    - **Severe loss of cognitive abilities**: inability to communicate, understand the environment, recognize loved ones.
    - **Physical decline**: muscular weakness, walking difficulties, incontinence, weight loss.
    - **Total dependence**: Requires assistance with all activities of daily living.

Diagnosing Alzheimer's disease

Diagnosis is based on a full clinical evaluation:

- **Medical interview**: medical history, symptom assessment, discussions with family and friends.
- **Cognitive tests**: Neuropsychological tests to assess memory, language, attention and visuospatial abilities.
- **Cerebral imaging**: CT or MRI scans to visualize brain structures, detect atrophy or rule out other pathologies.
- **Biological tests**: Blood tests to rule out other causes of dementia (vitamin deficiencies, thyroid disorders).

Early diagnosis means that interventions can be put in place to slow the progression of symptoms and improve quality of life.

Supporting people with Alzheimer's disease

Support is multidimensional, involving medical, psychosocial and environmental approaches.

1. **Medical care**

    - **Drug therapy**: use of acetylcholinesterase inhibitors (donepezil, rivastigmine) or memantine to slow the progression of cognitive symptoms.
    - **Management of associated symptoms**: Antidepressants, anxiolytics or antipsychotics to treat mood or behavior disorders, with caution due to side effects.
    - **Regular follow-up**: medical consultations to adjust treatments, monitor disease progression and manage comorbidities.

2. **Non-pharmacological interventions**

    - **Cognitive stimulation**: Activities designed to maintain cognitive functions, such as memory games, reading and puzzles.
    - **Occupational therapy**: Encouraging participation in meaningful activities adapted to the patient's abilities.

- **Reminiscence therapy**: Using past memories to stimulate recall and promote emotional well-being.
- **Music and art therapy**: Using music or art to improve mood, reduce anxiety and promote self-expression.

3. **Communication and relationships**

    - **Empathic approach**: Be patient, listen actively, respect the patient's rhythm.
    - **Simple communication**: Use short sentences, clear language, avoid complex questions.
    - **Emotional validation**: Acknowledging and accepting the emotions expressed, even if they seem incoherent.
    - **Maintaining eye contact and touch**: Encouraging emotional bonding, reassuring the patient.

4. **Adapting to the environment**

    - **Safety**: Install devices to prevent falls, and secure access to dangerous areas (kitchen, stairs).
    - **Simplicity**: Reduce distractions, organize space in an orderly fashion, use visual cues.
    - **Comfort**: Create a soothing environment, with familiar objects, photos and memories.
    - **Daily routine**: Establish regular schedules for meals, sleep and activities to reduce confusion.

5. **Support for activities of daily living**

    - **Progressive assistance**: Encourage patient autonomy by assisting only when necessary.
    - **Task adaptation**: Simplify complex activities, break tasks down into simple steps.

- **Use of technical aids**: adapted utensils, easy-to-wear clothing, devices to make it easier to take medication.

6. Psychosocial support

- **Support groups**: Participation in groups for patients and caregivers, enabling the sharing of experiences and strategies.
- **Intervention by professionals**: psychologists, social workers to support patients and their families in emotional and practical matters.

The role of caregivers and healthcare professionals

Caregivers, often family members, play a central role in supporting people with Alzheimer's disease. Their involvement can be a source of stress and exhaustion, so it's essential to support them:

- **Training**: Providing information on illness, communication techniques and managing difficult behavior.
- **Respite**: Offering solutions to relieve caregivers, such as homecare services and day-care centers.
- **Psychological support**: Offer consultations with professionals to deal with stress, depression or anxiety.

Healthcare professionals, including doctors, nurses, caregivers and occupational therapists, work as a team to provide comprehensive care:

- **Care coordination**: develop a personalized care plan, adapt interventions according to disease progression.
- **Interprofessional communication**: Sharing relevant information to ensure continuity of care.
- **Ongoing training**: Keep abreast of advances in the field to improve practices.

Legal and ethical aspects

Alzheimer's disease raises important questions about consent, decision-making capacity and legal protection:

- **Tutorship or guardianship**: Set up a legal protection measure if the patient is no longer able to manage his or her own affairs.
- **Advance directives**: Encourage patients to express their wishes regarding future care while they are still capable of doing so.
- **Respect for dignity**: Ensure that all interventions preserve the patient's integrity and fundamental rights.

Prevention and research

At present, there is no cure for Alzheimer's disease, but research continues to better understand the disease and develop new therapies. Certain measures can help reduce the risk or delay the onset of symptoms:

- **Regular physical activity**: Promotes cardiovascular and brain health.
- **Intellectual stimulation**: Continuous learning, social activities, cognitive games.
- **Balanced diet**: A diet rich in fruit, vegetables and fish, with a reduction in saturated fats.
- **Risk factor management**: control of hypertension, diabetes, cholesterol, smoking cessation.
-

- Dementia: types and non-drug approaches

Dementia is a syndrome characterized by a progressive and irreversible deterioration in cognitive functions, affecting memory, language, reasoning, behavior and the ability to carry out daily activities. It mainly affects the elderly, but can also occur in younger individuals. Understanding the different types of dementia and non-drug approaches to their management is essential to improving the quality of life of sufferers and their families. This presentation will explore the main types of dementia and non-pharmacological strategies for their management.

Understanding dementia

Dementia is not a disease in itself, but rather a set of symptoms resulting from various conditions affecting the brain. It manifests itself as an impairment of higher cognitive functions, interfering with social, professional and personal activities.

Types of dementia

1. **Alzheimer's disease**
    - **Description**: Alzheimer's disease is the most common form of dementia, accounting for 60-80% of cases. It is characterized by the formation of amyloid plaques and neurofibrillary tangles in the brain, leading to the death of neurons.
    - **Symptoms**: Progressive memory loss, language disorders, spatial and temporal disorientation, difficulty performing familiar tasks, mood and personality changes.

2. **Vascular dementia**
    - **Description**: Vascular dementia results from brain damage caused by blood circulation disorders, such as strokes or lacunar infarcts.
    - **Symptoms**: Sudden onset of cognitive problems, attention fluctuations, difficulty in planning and organizing, gait disorders, incontinence.

3. **Lewy body dementia**

    - **Description**: This form of dementia is caused by the presence of abnormal deposits of alpha-synuclein proteins (Lewy bodies) in neurons.
    - **Symptoms**: Cognitive fluctuations, recurrent visual hallucinations, REM sleep disorders, muscular rigidity, movement disorders similar to Parkinson's disease.

4. **Frontotemporal lobar degeneration**

    - **Description**: This dementia mainly affects the frontal and temporal lobes of the brain, responsible for behavior, personality and language.
    - **Symptoms**: Marked personality changes, inappropriate social behavior, apathy, language disorders (aphasia), difficulty understanding language.

5. **Dementia due to Parkinson's disease**

    - **Description**: Some people with Parkinson's disease develop dementia at an advanced stage.
    - **Symptoms**: Movement disorders (tremors, rigidity), cognitive slowdown, concentration difficulties, hallucinations.

6. **Mixed dementia**

    - **Description**: This is a combination of several types of dementia, usually Alzheimer's disease and vascular dementia.
    - **Symptoms**: Mixed clinical presentation, with symptoms characteristic of several types of dementia.

7. **Secondary dementias**

    ◦ **Description**: Some dementias are the result of underlying medical conditions such as vitamin deficiencies, thyroid disorders, infections or substance abuse.
    ◦ **Symptoms**: Variable, depending on the cause, with the possibility of improvement or reversibility if the cause is treated early.

Non-drug approaches to dementia

Non-pharmacological approaches play a crucial role in the care of people with dementia. They aim to improve quality of life, maintain autonomy, reduce behavioral and psychological symptoms, and support caregivers.

1. **Cognitive stimulation**

    ◦ **Objective**: Preserve and improve cognitive functions such as memory, attention, language and reasoning.
    ◦ **Methods** :
        - **Intellectual activities**: memory games, puzzles, crosswords, reading, discussions on a variety of subjects.
        - **Structured programs**: Cognitive therapies carried out by professionals, group sessions to stimulate cognitive abilities.

2. **Occupational therapies**

    ◦ **Objective**: Maintain involvement in daily activities, reinforce sense of usefulness and self-esteem.
    ◦ **Methods** :

- **Manual activities**: painting, gardening, cooking, DIY.
- **Task adaptation**: Simplify complex activities, use technical aids to facilitate task performance.

3. **Reminiscence therapy**

    - **Objective**: Evoke memories of the past to stimulate memory and promote emotional well-being.
    - **Methods** :
        - **Use of media**: photos, music, familiar objects, personal stories.
        - **Individual or group sessions**: Facilitator-led discussions to share memories and experiences.

4. **Music therapy**

    - **Objective**: Use music to improve mood, reduce anxiety and stimulate cognitive and motor functions.
    - **Methods** :
        - **Listening to music**: Selection of tunes enjoyed by the patient, songs from the past.
        - **Active participation**: Singing, playing simple instruments, moving in rhythm.

5. **Art therapy**

    - **Objective**: Encourage the expression of emotions and thoughts through artistic activities.
    - **Methods** :
        - **Creative activities**: drawing, painting, sculpture, collage.

- **Focus on the process**: Importance of commitment rather than artistic result.

6. **Animal therapy**

    - **Objective**: Improve emotional well-being, reduce stress and agitation through interaction with animals.
    - **Methods** :
        - **Animal visits**: Dogs, cats or other animals trained to interact with patients.
        - **Supervised activities**: Petting, feeding and playing with the animal under professional supervision.

7. **Physical exercise**

    - **Objective**: Maintain mobility, improve physical health, reduce depressive symptoms.
    - **Methods** :
        - **Adapted activities**: walking, tai chi, gentle gymnastics, swimming.
        - **Regular programs**: Sessions planned according to the patient's abilities.

8. **Behavioral approaches**

    - **Objective**: Manage behavioral and psychological symptoms such as agitation, aggression and wandering.
    - **Methods** :
        - **Identifying triggers**: Observe and understand the situations that lead to problem behaviors.
        - **Management strategies**: Adapt the environment, establish routines, use distraction or redirection.

9. **Snoezelen therapy**

    - **Objective**: Provide controlled sensory stimulation to soothe and relax the patient.
    - **Methods** :
        - **Multisensory environment**: Room equipped with soft lighting, soothing sounds, varied textures, pleasant aromas.
        - **Individualized sessions**: Accompanied by a therapist to adapt stimuli to the patient's preferences.

10. **Environmental interventions**

    - **Objective**: Adapt the living environment to reduce confusion and promote autonomy.
    - **Methods** :
        - **Clear signage**: use pictograms and colors to identify rooms or objects.
        - **Safety**: Installation of devices to prevent falls and restrict access to hazardous areas.
        - **Soothing layout**: Sober decoration, absence of visual or auditory overstimulation.

11. **Psychosocial support**

    - **Objective**: Offer emotional support, encourage social interaction, prevent isolation.
    - **Methods** :
        - **Support groups**: Meetings with other people with dementia or caregivers to share experiences.
        - **Social activities**: Participation in clubs, workshops and supervised outings.

The role of the caregiver in non-drug approaches

The caregiver plays a central role in the implementation of non-pharmacological approaches:

- **Careful observation**: Identify patient needs, preferences and reactions to adapt interventions.
- **Empathetic communication**: Use simple language, gestures, maintain eye contact, be patient.
- **Encouraging autonomy**: supporting patients in activities they can carry out on their own, rewarding their successes.
- **Behavior management** : Apply techniques to calm the patient in case of agitation, avoid confrontation.
- **Team collaboration**: Work closely with nurses, doctors, psychologists and occupational therapists.
- **Caregiver support**: Provide advice, share observations, refer to support resources.

Involving family members and caregivers

The role of loved ones is fundamental in supporting people with dementia:

- **Information and training**: Understanding the disease, symptoms and support strategies.
- **Participation in activities**: Involving family members in non-medication approaches to strengthen the emotional bond.
- **Self-care**: Encourage caregivers to take care of themselves and seek support to prevent burnout.

Ethics and respect for dignity

In all interventions, it is essential to respect the rights and dignity of people with dementia:

- **Consent**: Involve patients in decisions as much as possible, respect their choices.

- **Confidentiality**: Protect personal information, respect professional secrecy.
- **Individualized approach**: Tailor interventions to specific needs, avoid standardized solutions.

- Communication with disoriented patients

Communication with disoriented patients is a crucial aspect of care in geriatrics and psychiatry. People suffering from disorientation, whether temporary or chronic, experience an altered reality that can lead to anxiety, frustration and isolation. For healthcare professionals, establishing effective communication with these patients is essential to providing the necessary support, ensuring their safety and improving their quality of life. This article explores the challenges of communicating with disoriented patients and suggests approaches to fostering empathetic and constructive interaction.

Understanding disorientation

Disorientation manifests itself as confusion about time, space, personal identity or that of others. It can be caused by a variety of conditions, including dementia, Alzheimer's disease, neurological disorders, infections, metabolic imbalances or the side effects of certain medications. Disoriented patients may have difficulty understanding their environment, remembering recent events or recognizing familiar people. This confusion can lead to anxiety, agitation or maladaptive behavior.

The challenges of communication

Communicating with a disoriented person presents several challenges:

1. **Cognitive barriers**: problems with memory, attention and language can hamper comprehension and expression.

2. **Intense emotions**: Fear, frustration or agitation can make the patient less receptive to communication attempts.

3. **Misinterpretation**: The patient may misinterpret the caregiver's intentions, sometimes perceiving a threat where none exists.

4. **Variability of symptoms**: The degree of disorientation can fluctuate, making communication unpredictable.

Communication fundamentals

To establish effective communication with disoriented patients, several key principles must be adopted:

1. **Empathy and respect**: Put yourself in the patient's shoes, recognize their emotions and treat them with dignity.

2. **Patience**: Take the time needed, avoid showing impatience or frustration.

3. **Simplicity**: Use clear language, short sentences, avoid technical terms or complex metaphors.

4. **Consistency**: Maintain consistent routines and cues to reduce confusion.

5. **Positive non-verbal**: Adopt an open posture, a gentle tone of voice, soothing eye contact.

Effective communication techniques

1. **Calm, reassuring approach**
   Start every interaction by introducing yourself, even if the patient knows you. Use a calm, reassuring tone of voice. Avoid sudden movements or gestures that could be perceived as threatening.

2. **Using the patient's first name**
   Calling the patient by their first name can help capture their attention and establish a personal connection. It also reinforces their sense of identity.

3. **Simple, closed questions**
   Ask questions that require short answers or a simple "yes" or "no". Avoid overloading the patient with too much information at once.

4. **Active listening**
   Show that you are attentive to what the patient is expressing, verbally or non-verbally. Nod, repeat or rephrase to confirm your understanding.

5. **Validating feelings**
   Acknowledge the patient's emotions, even if you don't fully understand the source of their confusion. For example, "I can see you're worried, how can I help?"

6. **Use of visual aids**
   Images, familiar objects or visual cues can help the patient to better understand and situate himself. For example, show a clock to indicate mealtimes.

7. **Avoid confrontation**
   Do not directly contradict or correct the patient if he expresses false ideas. This can increase agitation. It's best to gently divert the conversation to a more soothing subject.

8. **Therapeutic touch**
   Light physical contact, such as holding hands or touching shoulders, can bring comfort if the patient is receptive. Make sure this gesture is appropriate and accepted.

9. **Reduce distractions**
   Create a calm environment to facilitate communication.

Turn off the TV or radio, avoid multiple conversations at the same time.

10. **Adapt your rhythm**

    Speak slowly, articulating clearly. Give the patient time to process the information and respond. Don't rush them.

Managing difficult behavior

Disoriented patients can sometimes show signs of agitation, aggression or opposition. Here are some strategies for dealing with these situations:

1. **Stay calm**

   Maintain a serene attitude. Your calmness can help soothe the patient.

2. **Identify triggers**

   Try to understand what may have triggered the behavior: pain, discomfort, fear, unmet need.

3. **Offering limited choices**

   Giving the patient a sense of control can reduce opposition. Offer simple options, for example, "Would you prefer orange juice or tea?"

4. **Use distraction**

   If the patient is fixated on a disturbing idea or behavior, suggest an alternative activity or subtly change the subject.

5. **Involving the family**

   Family members can provide valuable information about the patient's preferences and habits, helping to personalize the approach.

Importance of the environment

A suitable environment can greatly influence communication with disoriented patients:

- **Visual cues**: Use contrasting colors, pictograms or photos to make orientation easier.

- **Appropriate lighting**: Good lighting reduces shadows, which can be a source of confusion or fear.

- **Noise reduction**: Minimize sudden or loud noises that may disturb the patient.

- **Safety**: Make sure the area is safe to prevent accidents.

Staff training and support

Healthcare professionals must be trained to communicate effectively with disoriented patients:

- **Specialized training** : Participate in workshops or seminars on dementia, cognitive disorders and communication techniques.

- **Sharing experiences**: Exchange with colleagues on situations encountered and effective approaches.

- **Stress management**: taking care of your own mental health to avoid burnout.

Involving family and friends

The family plays a key role in supporting disoriented patients:

- **Regular communication**: Maintain contact with the patient through visits, calls and letters.

- **Information sharing**: Provide caregivers with details of the patient's habits, preferences and life history.

- **Emotional support**: offering comfort and love, essential to the patient's well-being.

Cardiovascular disorders

- Heart failure: monitoring and warning signs

Heart failure is a serious chronic condition characterized by the heart's inability to pump blood efficiently to meet the body's metabolic needs. The disease mainly affects the elderly, and represents a major public health issue due to its growing prevalence and impact on patients' quality of life. Careful monitoring and early detection of warning signs are essential to prevent complications, reduce hospitalization and improve prognosis. This paper explores key aspects of heart failure monitoring and identifies warning signs requiring medical intervention.

Understanding heart failure

Heart failure results from impaired cardiac function, due to a variety of underlying pathologies such as coronary artery disease, high blood pressure, cardiomyopathy or valvular heart disease. The weakened heart is no longer able to ensure adequate blood flow, leading to an accumulation of blood in the veins and congestion of the organs. The resulting symptoms have a considerable impact on patients' daily lives, and require comprehensive treatment.

Importance of monitoring

Regular monitoring of heart failure patients is crucial for :

- **Evaluating disease progression**: monitoring changes in health status helps to adapt treatment and prevent decompensation.

- **Detecting early signs of deterioration**: Early intervention can prevent hospitalization and serious complications.
- **Optimize treatment**: Adjust drug doses according to symptoms and clinical parameters.
- **Improving quality of life**: By reducing symptoms and preventing acute episodes, patients can maintain a more active, independent lifestyle.

Signs and symptoms of heart failure

The clinical manifestations of heart failure are varied and may include:

1. **Dyspnea**: Shortness of breath on exertion or at rest, aggravated when lying down (orthopnea) or at night (paroxysmal nocturnal dyspnea).
2. **Fatigue and weakness**: Decreased ability to perform daily activities due to insufficient oxygen supply to the muscles.
3. **Edema**: swelling of the lower limbs (ankles, legs), hands or abdomen (ascites) due to fluid retention.
4. **Rapid weight gain**: sudden weight gain due to fluid accumulation.
5. **Dry or productive cough**: sometimes accompanied by frothy sputum, especially when lying down.
6. **Palpitations**: sensation of rapid, irregular or strong heartbeat.
7. **Digestive disorders**: Loss of appetite, nausea, bloating due to liver and gastrointestinal congestion.
8. **Confusion or memory disorders**: reduced cerebral blood flow may affect cognitive function.

Monitoring patients with heart failure

Effective monitoring is based on several key elements:

1. **Body weight measurement**

    - **Significance**: Rapid weight gain may indicate fluid retention due to cardiac decompensation.
    - **Practical**: Weigh the patient daily, preferably in the morning after micturition and before breakfast, under similar conditions (light clothing, same scale).
    - **Interpretation**: An increase of more than 2 kg in 3 days should alert the caregiver.

2. **Assessment of respiratory symptoms**

    - **Observation of dyspnea**: Note onset or worsening of shortness of breath, need to sleep with several pillows, episodes of nocturnal coughing.
    - **Use of scales**: Dyspnea scales (such as the Borg scale) to quantify symptom intensity.

3. **Edema inspection**

    - **Location and extent**: Examine ankles, legs, sacrum in bedridden patients.
    - **Consistency**: press gently on the oedematous area to check for the presence of a bucket sign (imprint that persists for a few seconds).

4. **Blood pressure and pulse monitoring**

    - **Regular measurement**: Check blood pressure and heart rate for abnormalities.
    - **Heart rhythm**: Note irregularities, tachycardia or bradycardia.

5. **Diuresis assessment**

    o **Urine quantification**: monitor urine output, especially in patients on diuretics.
    o **Observation of color and frequency**: Signs of dehydration or associated renal failure.

6. **Monitoring general symptoms**

    o **Fatigue**: Note changes in energy levels, ability to perform usual activities.
    o **Appetite and digestion**: Monitor food intake, nausea and feelings of early satiety.
    o **Cognitive functions**: Observe signs of confusion, agitation and memory impairment.

Warning signs requiring medical intervention

Early recognition of signs of worsening heart failure is essential:

1. **Rapid weight gain**

    o **Significance**: Indicates fluid retention which may lead to pulmonary oedema.
    o **Action**: Contact physician to adjust diuretic therapy or assess clinical condition.

2. **Worsening dyspnea**

    o **Shortness of breath at rest**: inability to breathe comfortably even at rest.
    o **Nocturnal dyspnea**: frequent awakenings due to shortness of breath.
    o **Action**: Urgent medical consultation to assess the need for further treatment.

3. **Sudden or widespread edema**
    - **Rapid increase**: Appearance or worsening of edema in a short space of time.
    - **Action**: Inform doctor to adjust treatment.

4. **Chest pain**
    - **Angina**: oppressive chest pain that may indicate myocardial ischemia.
    - **Action**: Medical emergency, call emergency services.

5. **Palpitations or syncope**
    - **Rhythm disorders**: sensation of irregular heartbeat, malaise, loss of consciousness.
    - **Action**: Immediate medical assessment to rule out serious arrhythmia.

6. **Mental confusion**
    - **Abrupt change**: disorientation, disturbances of consciousness which may indicate cerebral hypoxia.
    - **Action**: Rapid medical intervention to determine the cause.

7. **Marked reduction in diuresis**
    - **Oliguria**: significant decrease in urine production, possible sign of acute renal failure.
    - **Action**: Medical consultation to assess renal function and adjust treatment.

Role of the caregiver in monitoring and management

The caregiver is in a privileged position to observe and report changes in the patient's condition:

1. **Careful observation**

    - **Clinical signs**: Note changes in symptoms and the appearance of new signs.
    - **Behavior**: Observe changes in mood, appetite, activity level.

2. **Effective communication**

    - **Transmissions**: Inform the nurse or doctor of relevant observations.
    - **Documentation**: Record monitoring data in the patient's file.

3. **Patient education**

    - **Information on the disease**: Explain the symptoms to watch out for and the importance of taking medication regularly.
    - **Practical advice**: Encourage daily weighing, a suitable diet (sodium restriction) and moderate physical activity.

4. **Psychological support**

    - **Active listening**: Allowing patients to express their concerns and feelings.
    - **Motivation**: Encourage compliance, reward patient efforts.

5. **Preventing complications**

    - **Fluid watch**: Monitor fluid intake as prescribed.
    - **Infection prevention**: Encourage rigorous hygiene to avoid respiratory superinfections.

Collaboration with the multidisciplinary team

- **Nurses**: Share observations, participate in technical care (administering medication, monitoring vital signs).
- **Doctors**: Inform about warning signs, help adjust care plan.
- **Dieticians**: Collaborate to adapt the patient's diet (low-salt diet, nutritional balance).
- **Physiotherapists**: Facilitate exercise rehabilitation and breathing exercises.

Complementary approaches to improving quality of life

- **Adapted physical activity**: Encourage moderate exercise to strengthen cardiac capacity, under medical supervision.
- **Stress management**: relaxation techniques, psychological support to reduce illness-related anxiety.
- **Stop smoking and limit alcohol consumption**: Tips for adopting a healthy lifestyle and reducing aggravating factors.

- Hypertension: preventive measures

Hypertension, often dubbed the "silent killer", is a chronic condition characterized by excessively high blood pressure in the arteries. It is one of the world's leading causes of cardiovascular disease, stroke and kidney failure. Despite its major impact on public health, it often remains unrecognized or neglected, as it can evolve without apparent symptoms for many years. Prevention of hypertension is therefore essential to reduce the associated morbidity and mortality. This article explores effective preventive measures to combat this condition.

Understanding hypertension

Blood pressure is the force exerted by blood on the artery walls during circulation. It is determined by two measurements:

1. **Systolic pressure**: pressure during heart contraction (systole).
2. **Diastolic pressure**: pressure when the heart relaxes between beats (diastole).

Normal blood pressure is generally less than 120/80 mmHg. Hypertension is diagnosed when systolic pressure is equal to or greater than 140 mmHg and/or diastolic pressure is equal to or greater than 90 mmHg, on repeated measurements.

The importance of prevention

Preventing hypertension is crucial for several reasons:

- **Reduced cardiovascular risk**: Hypertension increases the risk of heart disease, stroke and heart failure.
- **Preserving kidney health**: High pressure can damage the kidneys, leading to kidney failure.
- **Improved quality of life**: Preventing hypertension helps maintain good general health and avoid long-term complications.

Risk factors for hypertension

Understanding risk factors is essential to implementing effective preventive measures. Risk factors can be divided into two categories: non-modifiable and modifiable.

1. **Non-modifiable factors**
    - **Age**: The risk of hypertension increases with age, due to the loss of elasticity in the arteries.
    - **Heredity**: A family history of hypertension increases individual risk.

- **Gender**: Men are generally more at risk before the age of 55, while women are more at risk after the menopause.

2. **Modifiable factors**

    - **Sedentary lifestyle**: Lack of physical activity encourages overweight and hypertension.
    - **High-salt diet**: Excessive sodium consumption contributes to high blood pressure.
    - **Excessive alcohol consumption**: Alcohol abuse can raise blood pressure.
    - **Overweight and obesity**: Excess weight puts extra strain on the heart.
    - **Smoking**: nicotine and other tobacco chemicals damage arterial walls.
    - **Stress**: Chronic stress can have a negative impact on blood pressure.

Measures to prevent hypertension

The key to prevention lies in adopting a healthy, active lifestyle. Here are the main measures to take:

1. **Adopt a balanced diet**

    - **Reduce salt intake**: Limit sodium intake to less than 5 grams a day (about one teaspoon). This means cutting down on processed foods, deli meats, salty cheeses and ready-made meals.
    - **Increase consumption of fruit and vegetables**: Rich in potassium, fibre and antioxidants, they help regulate blood pressure.
    - **Choose whole grains**: Whole grains promote cardiovascular health.
    - **Limit saturated and trans fats**: Reduce consumption of fatty meats, full-fat dairy products, fried foods and industrial pastries.

- **Adopt the DASH** (*Dietary Approaches to Stop Hypertension*) **diet**: This diet recommends a diet rich in fruits, vegetables, low-fat dairy products, whole grains, poultry, fish and nuts, while limiting fats, red meats and added sugars.

2. **Maintaining a healthy weight**

    - **Calculating body mass index (BMI)**: A BMI between 18.5 and 24.9 is considered normal.
    - **Progressive weight loss**: In cases of overweight or obesity, moderate weight loss (5-10% of body weight) can significantly reduce blood pressure.
    - **Balancing calorie intake and energy expenditure**: adapting diet and physical activity to maintain a stable weight.

3. **Regular physical activity**

    - **Recommendations**: At least 150 minutes of moderate-intensity aerobic activity per week (for example, 30 minutes a day, 5 days a week).
    - **Types of activity**: Brisk walking, swimming, cycling, dancing, jogging.
    - **Muscle strengthening**: Incorporate strength training twice a week to improve overall health.

4. **Limiting alcohol consumption**

    - **Recommendations**: No more than two standard drinks a day for men and one for women, with at least two alcohol-free days a week.
    - **Understanding units**: A standard glass corresponds to about 10 grams of pure alcohol (e.g. 250 ml of 5% beer, 100 ml of 12% wine, 30 ml of 40% spirits).

5. **Quitting smoking**

    - **Effects of tobacco**: Nicotine raises blood pressure and accelerates heart rate. The chemicals in tobacco damage artery walls, promoting atherosclerosis.
    - **Withdrawal strategies**: Consult a health professional, use nicotine substitutes, participate in smoking cessation programs.

6. **Managing stress**

    - **Relaxation techniques**: yoga, meditation, deep breathing, tai chi.
    - **Relaxing activities**: Reading, music, arts and crafts, nature walks.
    - **Work/life balance**: taking time for yourself, avoiding work overload.

7. **Limit caffeine consumption**

    - **Effect on blood pressure**: Caffeine may cause a temporary rise in blood pressure in some people.
    - **Recommendations**: Consume in moderation, observe your own sensitivity.

8. **Monitor blood pressure regularly**

    - **Self-measurement at home**: using a validated blood pressure monitor to track blood pressure.
    - **Regular consultations**: Visits to the doctor for professional follow-up, especially in the presence of risk factors.

9. **Limiting exposure to pollution**

    ○ **Effects of pollution**: Fine particles can contribute to hypertension by damaging blood vessels.
    ○ **Precautions**: Avoid high-pollution areas, especially during peak periods, and prefer green spaces.

10. **Inform and educate**

    ○ **Know the risk factors**: Understand the importance of each preventive measure.
    ○ **Participate in educational programs**: Workshops, conferences, information sessions on cardiovascular health.

The role of healthcare professionals in prevention

Doctors, nurses, pharmacists and other healthcare professionals play an essential role in preventing high blood pressure:

- **Individual risk assessment**: Identification of risk factors specific to each individual.
- **Personalized advice**: Development of a tailored prevention plan, including recommendations on diet, physical activity and lifestyle.
- **Regular follow-up**: Monitor blood pressure, adjust advice according to progress.
- **Compliance support**: Encouragement to maintain lifestyle changes, help to overcome obstacles.

Involvement of the community and health policies

Preventing hypertension also requires action at community and national level:

- **Awareness programs**: Information campaigns on the risks of hypertension and how to prevent it.
- **Promoting physical activity**: Designing public spaces to encourage exercise (parks, bike paths, sports facilities).
- **Food regulations**: reduction of salt content in processed foods, clear product labelling.
- **Access to care**: Facilitate access to health services for screening and monitoring hypertension.

- Stroke: post-stroke management

Stroke is a major medical emergency that occurs when blood flow to a part of the brain is interrupted, causing brain cells to die. Stroke is a major cause of death and disability worldwide. Stroke management is crucial to maximize the chances of recovery, prevent recurrence and improve patients' quality of life. This article explores the different facets of post-stroke management, emphasizing the importance of a multidisciplinary, patient-centered approach.

Understanding stroke

There are two main types of stroke:

1. **Ischemic stroke**: Accounts for around 85% of cases, and is caused by a blood clot blocking a cerebral artery, leading to a reduction or cessation of blood supply to part of the brain.

2. **Hemorrhagic stroke**: Occurs when a cerebral blood vessel ruptures, causing hemorrhage into the brain. This

may be due to uncontrolled high blood pressure or vascular malformation.

Symptoms of stroke can include sudden weakness or numbness on one side of the body, impaired speech or understanding, vision loss, severe headaches or sudden confusion.

The importance of post-stroke management

The period following a stroke is critical for the patient. Proper management can :

- **Improve functional recovery**: Reduce motor, sensory and cognitive deficits.
- **Prevent complications**: avoid infections, pressure sores, swallowing disorders or deep vein thrombosis.
- **Reduce the risk of recidivism**: Implement measures to control risk factors.
- **Supporting patients and their families**: offering psychological and social support to help them cope with life changes.

Stages of post-stroke management

1. **Acute hospital phase**
   - **Medical stabilization**: monitoring vital signs, controlling blood pressure, managing immediate complications.
   - **Initial assessment**: Neurological examinations, brain imaging (CT scan, MRI) to determine type and extent of stroke.
   - **Specific treatments** :
     - *Ischemic stroke*: Intravenous thrombolysis to dissolve the clot, mechanical thrombectomy to remove the clot.

- *Hemorrhagic stroke*: Control of hypertension, surgical interventions to evacuate hematoma or repair vessels.

2. **Early inpatient rehabilitation**

    - **Early mobilization**: Prevention of complications associated with immobility (bedsores, pulmonary embolism).
    - **Multidisciplinary assessment**: motor, cognitive, language, swallowing and emotional functions.
    - **Start of rehabilitation**:
        - *Physiotherapy*: Exercises to improve muscle strength, balance and coordination.
        - *Speech therapy*: Language and swallowing rehabilitation.
        - *Occupational therapy*: Learning or relearning activities of daily living.

3. **Rehabilitation in a specialized center or at home**

    - **Personalized rehabilitation program**: Tailored to the patient's specific needs, with realistic, progressive objectives.
    - **Professional presentations**:
        - *Physiotherapists*: Motor therapies, gait rehabilitation.
        - *Speech therapists*: Improving communication, swallowing exercises.
        - *Occupational therapists*: Adapting the environment, using technical aids.
        - *Neuropsychologists*: Cognitive support, management of attention and memory disorders.
        - *Social assistants*: help in organizing the return home, administrative procedures.

4. **Secondary prevention**

    ○ **Controlling risk factors** :
    - *Hypertension*: Regular monitoring, antihypertensive treatment.
    - *Diabetes*: Glycemic control, adapted diet.
    - *Hypercholesterolemia*: Lipid-lowering diet, statins.
    - *Smoking*: Stop smoking, cessation programs.
    - *Sedentary lifestyle*: Encourage regular physical activity.

    ○ **Drug treatments** :
    - *Antiplatelet agents*: Aspirin, clopidogrel to prevent the formation of new clots.
    - *Anticoagulants* : In case of atrial fibrillation or other cardiac rhythm disorders.

    ○ **Regular medical follow-up**: Consultations with neurologist, cardiologist and GP.

5. **Psychological and social support**

    ○ **Managing emotional disorders**: Depression, anxiety and irritability are common after a stroke.
    ○ **Psychological therapy**: Psychologists and psychiatrists help patients adapt to change.
    ○ **Support groups**: meetings with other patients to share experiences and break isolation.
    ○ **Family involvement**: Support for caregivers, information on the disease, advice on day-to-day support.

Functional rehabilitation

Rehabilitation is a central component of post-stroke care. It aims to :

- **Restoring lost capacities**: Through cerebral plasticity, the brain can reorganize its neural networks.
- **Compensating for deficits**: Learning alternative strategies for performing tasks.
- **Prevention of secondary complications**: muscular contractures, musculoskeletal disorders.

Rehabilitation strategies

1. **Motor rehabilitation**

    - **Active exercises**: Mobilization of affected limbs to strengthen muscles.
    - **Induced constraint therapy**: Immobilization of the healthy limb to encourage use of the affected limb.
    - **Assistive technologies**: rehabilitation robots, virtual reality to stimulate patient involvement.

2. **Language rehabilitation**

    - **Oral expression exercises**: Pronunciation, sentence formation.
    - **Comprehension**: Work on understanding instructions and texts.
    - **Alternative communication**: use of gestures, pictograms, tablets.

3. **Cognitive rehabilitation**

    - **Memory exercises**: memory games, information recall.
    - **Attention and concentration**: Targeted tasks to improve focus.
    - **Executive functions**: planning, organization, problem solving.

4. **Swallowing rehabilitation**

    - **Compensation techniques**: Specific positions to facilitate swallowing.
    - **Diet adaptation**: modified textures, thickened liquids to prevent false routes.
    - **Muscle exercises**: Strengthening swallowing muscles.

Adapting the environment and returning home

1. **Home improvements**

    - **Accessibility**: Removing obstacles, installing ramps, widening doorways.
    - **Safety**: Grab bars in the bathroom, non-slip floors.
    - **Technical aids**: wheelchairs, walkers, patient lifts.

2. **Home help**

    - **Assistance services**: caregivers, personal care assistants.
    - **Domestic support**: help with household chores, shopping and meal preparation.
    - **Teleassistance**: Alert systems in the event of a fall or medical emergency.

Resuming social and professional activities

- **Social reintegration**: Participation in community activities, adapted leisure activities.
- **Returning to work**: assessment of abilities, adaptation of workstation, part-time therapy.
- **Driving**: Medical assessment to determine fitness to drive, specific training if necessary.

Recurrence prevention

Secondary prevention is essential to reduce the risk of another stroke:

- **Adherence to treatment** : Regular use of prescribed medication.

- **Healthy lifestyle**:
    - *Balanced diet*: rich in fruit, vegetables and fish, low in saturated fats and salt.
    - *Physical activity*: Regular exercise adapted to the patient's abilities.
    - *Smoking cessation*: Avoid active and passive smoking.
    - *Moderate alcohol consumption*: Limit alcohol according to medical recommendations.

- **Medical monitoring**: Regular checks of blood pressure, cholesterol and blood sugar levels.

Support for caregivers

Relatives play a crucial role in post-stroke care, but can face significant stress:

- **Information and training**: Understanding the nature of stroke, patient needs, care techniques.
- **Emotional support**: discussion groups, psychological support to deal with exhaustion and depression.
- **External resources**: Turning to associations and social services for help.

Innovation and research

Research continues to bring new perspectives to stroke management:

- **Innovative therapies**: Stem cells, neurostimulation, gene therapies under evaluation.
- **Rehabilitation technologies**: Exoskeletons, brain-machine interfaces to improve motor recovery.
- **Telemedicine programs**: remote monitoring, online consultations for rural areas or patients with reduced mobility.

Respiratory conditions

- Chronic obstructive pulmonary disease (COPD)

Chronic obstructive pulmonary disease (COPD) is a chronic respiratory disease characterized by progressive and irreversible obstruction of the airways, resulting in restricted respiratory flow. The condition encompasses two main pathologies: chronic bronchitis and pulmonary emphysema. COPD is a major cause of morbidity and mortality worldwide, affecting millions of people and representing a major public health issue. Understanding the mechanisms, risk factors, symptoms, diagnosis and management of COPD is essential to improving patients' quality of life and reducing the impact of the disease.

Pathophysiology of COPD

COPD results from chronic inflammation of the airways and lung parenchyma, leading to structural alterations :

1. **Chronic bronchitis**: Inflammation and thickening of the bronchial mucosa, with hyperproduction of mucus, leading to a persistent, productive cough.

2. **Pulmonary emphysema**: Destruction of alveolar walls, loss of pulmonary elasticity, leading to hyperinflation of the lungs and reduced gas exchange.

These changes result in airway obstruction, expiratory flow limitation and inefficient ventilation, leading to hypoxemia (reduced oxygen in the blood) and, in advanced cases, hypercapnia (increased carbon dioxide in the blood).

Risk factors and causes

COPD is a multifactorial disease, in which environmental and genetic factors interact:

1. **Smoking**: The main risk factor. Cigarette smoke contains toxic substances that cause inflammation and damage to the respiratory tract.

2. **Occupational exposure**: Prolonged inhalation of dusts, fumes or chemicals in certain occupations (miners, construction workers, textile workers).

3. **Air pollution**: Exposure to outdoor pollutants (nitrogen dioxide, fine particles) and indoor pollutants (biomass smoke for cooking or heating).

4. **Genetic factors**: Deficiency of alpha-1 antitrypsin, a protein that protects the lungs from destructive enzymes.

5. **Repeated respiratory infections**: Especially in childhood, these can affect lung development.

6. **Low socio-economic status**: associated with increased exposure to risk factors and limited access to care.

Symptoms and clinical manifestations

COPD develops slowly, and symptoms usually appear after years of silent progression:

1. **Chronic cough**: Often referred to as "smoker's cough", it is productive, with mucous or mucopurulent sputum.

2. **Dyspnea**: Shortness of breath on exertion, then at rest in advanced stages, due to airflow limitation.

3. **Wheezing and rales**: Audible respiratory sounds associated with airway obstruction.

4. **Chest tightness**: Sensation of tight or heavy chest.

5. **Fatigue**: due to increased breathing effort and tissue hypoxia.

6. **Weight loss**: In advanced stages, due to increased energy expenditure and anorexia.

7. **Exacerbations**: Acute episodes of worsening symptoms, often triggered by respiratory infections.

Diagnosis of COPD

Early diagnosis is crucial to slowing the progression of the disease:

1. **Anamnesis**: Detailed questioning about symptoms, smoking history and occupational exposure.

2. **Clinical examination**: Pulmonary auscultation to detect rales, wheezing, prolonged expiratory time.

3. **Spirometry**: the benchmark respiratory function test, measuring lung volumes and expiratory flows. FEV1 (forced expiratory volume in seconds) and FEV1/CV (vital capacity) are reduced in COPD.

4. **Chest X-ray**: may show signs of emphysema, pulmonary hyperinflation, flattening of the diaphragmatic cupolas.

5. **Blood gases**: Assess gas exchange, look for hypoxemia and hypercapnia.

6. **Alpha-1 antitrypsin assay**: Especially in young patients or non-smokers, to detect a genetic deficiency.

7. **Exercise tests**: Assessment of exercise tolerance and oxygen desaturation.

Severity classification

The severity of COPD is classified according to the criteria of the Global Initiative for Chronic Obstructive Lung Disease (GOLD):

- **GOLD 1 (mild)**: FEV1 ≥ 80% of predicted value.
- **GOLD 2 (moderate)** : FEV1 between 50% and 79%.
- **GOLD 3 (severe)**: FEV1 between 30% and 49%.
- **GOLD 4 (very severe)**: FEV1 < 30%.

This classification also takes into account symptoms and exacerbations to guide treatment.

COPD management

COPD management aims to relieve symptoms, improve quality of life, slow disease progression and prevent exacerbations:

1. **Smoking cessation**
   - **Most effective measure**: Smoking cessation slows the decline in lung function.
   - **Support**: Behavioural therapies, nicotine substitutes, medications (varenicline, bupropion).

2. **Pharmacological treatments**
   - **Inhaled bronchodilators**: basic medications for relieving dyspnea.

- - **Short-acting beta-2 agonists (SABA)**: Rapid relief of symptoms.
  - **Long-acting beta-2 agonists (LABA)**: Prolonged symptom control.
  - **Anticholinergics**: reduce bronchial tone, available in short-acting (SAMA) and long-acting (LAMA) forms.
  - **Inhaled corticosteroids**: reduce inflammation, indicated for patients with frequent exacerbations.
  - **Combination therapy**: A combination of bronchodilators and corticosteroids for enhanced efficacy.
  - **Theophylline**: Oral bronchodilator, less widely used because of side effects.
  - **Phosphodiesterase-4 inhibitors**: For patients with chronic bronchitis and frequent exacerbations.

3. **Oxygen therapy**

   - **Indication**: For patients with severe hypoxemia ($PaO_2 \leq 55$ mmHg).
   - **Goal**: Improve survival, reduce polycythemia, relieve dyspnea.
   - **Modalities**: Long-term oxygen therapy (at least 15 hours a day).

4. **Respiratory rehabilitation**

   - **Multidisciplinary program**: physical exercise, education, nutritional support, behavioral therapy.
   - **Objectives**: Improve exercise tolerance, reduce dyspnea, improve quality of life.

5. **Vaccinations**

    ◦ **Flu vaccine**: Annual, to prevent respiratory infections.
    ◦ **Pneumococcal vaccine**: Protection against bacterial pneumonia.

6. **Exacerbation management**

    ◦ **Treatment of infections** : Antibiotics in cases of suspected bacterial infection.
    ◦ **Systemic corticosteroids**: Reduce inflammation during severe exacerbations.
    ◦ **Short-acting bronchodilators**: increase dose or frequency.

7. **Surgical procedures**

    ◦ **Lung volume reduction surgery**: resection of emphysematous areas to improve respiratory function.
    ◦ **Lung transplantation**: For young patients with very severe COPD.

Patient education and support

1. **Therapeutic education**

    ◦ **Knowledge of the disease**: understanding symptoms, treatments, signs of exacerbation.
    ◦ **Self-management**: learning correct inhalation techniques, compliance with treatment.

2. **Psychological support**

    ◦ **Anxiety and depression**: Frequent in COPD patients, requiring appropriate support.

- **Support groups**: sharing experiences, boosting motivation to quit smoking and adherence to treatment.

3. **Nutritional advice**

    - **Overweight**: Can aggravate dyspnea, requires dietary management.
    - **Denutrition**: Frequent in the advanced stages, requiring appropriate caloric intake.

Prevention and screening

1. **Primary prevention**

    - **Tobacco control**: public health policies, smoking bans in public places, taxation.
    - **Reducing occupational exposure**: Safety standards, personal protective equipment.

2. **Early detection**

    - **Population at risk**: Smokers or ex-smokers over 40, people exposed to harmful agents.
    - **Screening spirometry**: To detect airway obstruction before symptoms appear.

Socio-economic impact of COPD

- **High cost of care**: frequent hospitalization, long-term treatment.
- **Loss of productivity**: work stoppages, disability.
- **Burden on families**: Support for dependent patients, psychological impact.

Research and future prospects

1. **New therapies**

    ◦ **Drugs targeting inflammation**: cytokine inhibitors, monoclonal antibodies.
    ◦ **Regenerative therapies**: stem cells to repair damaged lung tissue.

2. **Customized approaches**

    ◦ **Patient phenotyping**: Treatments adapted to individual characteristics.
    ◦ **Biomarkers**: To predict response to treatment and disease progression.

3. **Digital technologies**

    ◦ **Telemedicine**: remote patient monitoring, early detection of exacerbations.
    ◦ **Mobile applications**: self-management tools, medication reminders, symptom recording.

- Pneumonia: prevention and care

Pneumonia is an acute infection of lung tissue, mainly affecting the alveoli where the gas exchange essential for breathing takes place. It is caused by a variety of micro-organisms, including bacteria, viruses and fungi. Pneumonia is a major global health problem, particularly affecting young children, the elderly and individuals with weakened immune systems. Understanding the mechanisms of this disease, prevention methods and care approaches is essential to reduce its prevalence and potentially serious consequences.

Understanding pneumonia

Pneumonia is characterized by inflammation of the pulmonary alveoli, often accompanied by filling of the alveoli with fluid or pus. This accumulation impairs blood oxygenation, leading to significant respiratory symptoms and, in severe cases, respiratory distress.

Causes and risk factors

1. **Infectious agents** :

    - **Bacteria**: *Streptococcus pneumoniae* (pneumococcus) is the most common bacterial cause in adults. Other bacteria, such as *Haemophilus influenzae*, *Staphylococcus aureus* and certain Gram-negative bacilli, may also be involved.
    - **Viruses**: Respiratory viruses such as influenza, respiratory syncytial virus (RSV) and coronavirus can cause viral pneumonia.
    - **Fungi**: Fungi such as *Pneumocystis* jirovecii can cause pneumonia in immunocompromised people.

2. **Risk factors** :

    - **Advanced age**: People over 65 are more likely to develop pneumonia due to a weakened immune system.
    - **Young children**: Children's immature immune systems make them vulnerable.
    - **Chronic diseases**: conditions such as diabetes, heart failure or COPD increase the risk.
    - **Smoking**: Tobacco damages the respiratory tract and reduces lung defenses.
    - **Alcoholism**: Alcohol abuse can weaken the immune system and increase the risk of aspiration.
    - **Immune deficiency**: Patients undergoing chemotherapy or living with HIV/AIDS are at greater risk.

- **Hospitalization**: Hospitalized patients, especially those in intensive care, are at risk of nosocomial pneumonia.

Symptoms and clinical manifestations

Symptoms of pneumonia can vary depending on the causative agent, the patient's age and general state of health. Common manifestations include:

- **Fever**: often high, accompanied by chills.
- **Cough**: Initially dry, then productive with purulent expectoration.
- **Dyspnea**: Shortness of breath, difficulty breathing.
- **Chest pain**: acute pain, often increased by deep breathing or coughing.
- **Fatigue**: Feeling of general weakness and malaise.
- **Mental confusion**: Particularly in the elderly, may indicate severe infection.
- **Tachypnea**: Rapid, shallow breathing.
- **Tachycardia**: Elevated heart rate in response to infection.

Diagnosis of pneumonia

Accurate diagnosis is essential for effective management:

1. **Anamnesis and clinical examination** :
   - **Interrogatory**: Collection of symptoms, duration, aggravating or mitigating factors, medical history.
   - **Pulmonary auscultation**: Detection of abnormal noises such as crackles or bronchial rales.

2. **Additional tests** :

    - **Chest X-ray**: Visualization of pulmonary infiltrates characteristic of pneumonia.
    - **Blood tests**: CBC to detect leukocytosis, elevated inflammatory markers (CRP, procalcitonin).
    - **Blood gases**: Assessment of blood oxygenation and acid-base balance.
    - **Sputum examination**: culture and antibiotic susceptibility test to identify the pathogen and determine antibiotic sensitivity.
    - **Hemocultures**: Testing for bacteria in blood in cases of suspected septicemia.

Pneumonia treatment and care

Therapeutic management depends on the severity of the pneumonia, the presumed or identified causative agent, and the patient's characteristics.

1. **Antibiotic treatments** :

    - **Bacterial pneumonia**: Prescription of appropriate antibiotics. In the absence of precise identification, empirical treatment targeting the most likely germs is initiated.
    - **Treatment adjustment** : Adjustment according to antibiogram results and clinical evolution.

2. **Antiviral treatments** :

    - **Viral pneumonia**: Administration of specific antivirals whenever possible (e.g. oseltamivir for influenza). Treatment is often symptomatic.

3. **Supportive care** :

    - **Oxygen therapy**: Administration of oxygen to correct hypoxemia.
    - **Hydration**: Maintain adequate hydration to thin bronchial secretions.
    - **Antipyretics and analgesics**: Paracetamol to reduce fever and relieve pain.
    - **Respiratory physiotherapy**: Helps evacuate secretions and improve ventilation.

4. **Hospitalization** :

    - **Hospitalization criteria**: severe pneumonia, comorbidities, advanced age, inability to take oral medication, respiratory distress.
    - **Intensive care** : For patients with acute respiratory failure or hemodynamic instability.

5. **Monitoring and follow-up** :

    - **Regular clinical assessment**: monitoring of vital signs, oxygen saturation, response to treatment.
    - **Radiological re-evaluation**: If symptoms persist or worsen, or to confirm resolution of infection.

Pneumonia prevention

Prevention is the key to reducing the incidence of pneumonia, particularly in at-risk populations.

1. **Vaccinations** :

    - **Pneumococcal vaccine**: Recommended for children, people over 65, and individuals at risk (chronic illness, immunosuppression).
    - **Flu vaccine**: Annual vaccination to prevent influenza, which can predispose to pneumonia.

- **Other vaccines**: *Haemophilus influenzae* type b (Hib) vaccination for children.

2. **Personal and collective hygiene :**

    - **Hand washing**: Regular and thorough, especially after coughing or sneezing.
    - **Respiratory etiquette**: Cover mouth and nose with a handkerchief or elbow when coughing or sneezing.
    - **Isolation of infected persons**: Limit the spread of respiratory infections.

3. **Healthy lifestyle:**

    - **Smoking cessation**: Reduced airway damage and improved lung defences.
    - **Balanced diet**: sufficient intake of essential nutrients to support the immune system.
    - **Regular physical activity**: strengthens the body's defenses and improves lung capacity.

4. **Protecting vulnerable populations :**

    - **Increased surveillance**: For the elderly and immunocompromised patients, with particular attention to the first signs of infection.
    - **Health education**: Raising awareness of preventive measures and the importance of seeking prompt medical attention in the event of symptoms.

The role of healthcare professionals in prevention and care

1. **Education and awareness :**

    - **Patient information**: On risk factors, warning signs and preventive measures.

- **Promoting vaccination**: Encouraging and facilitating access to recommended vaccines.

2. **Early screening and diagnosis** :
   - **Rapid recognition of symptoms**: to initiate appropriate treatment without delay.
   - **Judicious use of complementary tests**: To confirm diagnosis and guide treatment.

3. **Therapeutic management** :
   - **Appropriate prescribing**: Choice of antibiotics based on recommendations and local resistance.
   - **Monitoring treatment efficacy**: Adjust if necessary according to clinical evolution.

4. **Prevention of nosocomial infections** :
   - **Compliance with hygiene protocols**: hand washing, use of personal protective equipment.
   - **Ongoing training**: Regular updates on best practices.

Possible complications of pneumonia

Pneumonia can lead to complications, especially if not treated promptly or in frail patients:

- **Pleural effusion**: accumulation of fluid in the pleural cavity, which may require puncture.
- **Pleural empyema**: collection of pus in the pleural cavity, requiring drainage.
- **Pulmonary abscess**: Formation of purulent cavities in lung tissue.
- **Bacteremia**: Spread of infection in the bloodstream, leading to septicemia.

- **Acute respiratory failure**: requiring ventilatory support.
- **Acute respiratory distress syndrome (ARDS)**: Diffuse inflammation of the lungs, severely compromising oxygenation.

- Use of oxygen therapy

Oxygen therapy is a therapeutic method involving the administration of oxygen to patients suffering from hypoxemia, i.e. insufficient oxygen in the blood. The aim is to improve oxygen supply to the tissues and organs essential for optimal body function. Oxygen therapy is a key component in the management of many respiratory and cardiovascular conditions, and its appropriate use can significantly improve patients' quality of life and prognosis.

Oxygen is essential to life. Every cell in the body needs it to produce the energy required for its metabolic functions, through the process of cellular respiration. When oxygen supply is compromised, cells can no longer function properly, leading to organ dysfunction and, in severe cases, multi-organ failure. Tissue hypoxia can result from a variety of pathological conditions, including lung or heart disease, or acute situations such as poisoning.

Oxygen therapy indications

Oxygen therapy is indicated in several clinical situations where oxygenation is impaired:

1. **Chronic lung disease**: patients with chronic obstructive pulmonary disease (COPD), emphysema or pulmonary fibrosis may present with chronic hypoxemia requiring long-term oxygen therapy.

2. **Acute respiratory failure**: In conditions such as pneumonia, pulmonary edema, severe asthma or acute

respiratory distress syndrome (ARDS), oxygen therapy is essential to correct hypoxemia.

3. **Cardiovascular disorders**: congestive heart failure may result in poor oxygenation due to insufficient blood flow, justifying the use of oxygen.

4. **Emergency situations**: In the event of myocardial infarction, shock, massive hemorrhage or carbon monoxide poisoning, oxygen administration is crucial.

5. **Severe anemia**: Although less common, profound anemia may require oxygen therapy to ensure adequate tissue oxygenation.

Methods of administration

Oxygen can be administered in a variety of ways, depending on the patient's needs, the level of hypoxemia and the clinical context:

1. **Nasal cannula (oxygen spectacles)**: This is a simple device consisting of two small tubes inserted into the nostrils. It delivers oxygen at a low flow rate (1 to 6 liters per minute), ideal for patients requiring a moderate supply of oxygen while retaining a certain degree of comfort and the ability to speak and eat.

2. **Single face mask**: This mask covers the nose and mouth, allowing a higher flow of oxygen (5 to 10 liters per minute). It is used when oxygen needs are greater than can be provided by the nasal cannula.

3. **Reservoir mask (high-concentration mask)**: Equipped with a reservoir bag, it can deliver high oxygen concentrations (up to 90-95%) at flow rates of 10 to 15 liters per minute. It is indicated in situations of severe hypoxemia.

4. **Venturi mask**: This device delivers a precise concentration of oxygen, thanks to a system of calibrated valves. It is particularly useful for COPD patients, in whom hyperoxia can be deleterious.

5. **High-flow oxygen therapy**: Used in intensive care, this delivers heated and humidified oxygen at very high flow rates (up to 60 liters per minute), improving the comfort and efficiency of ventilation.

6. **Non-invasive ventilation**: For patients in acute respiratory failure, the addition of positive pressure can help keep the airways open and improve oxygenation.

Precautions and monitoring

Oxygen administration, although life-saving, requires careful monitoring to avoid potential complications:

- **Hyperoxia**: Excessive oxygen intake can lead to toxicity, particularly in the lungs and retina of neonates. In COPD patients, too high a concentration of oxygen can suppress the respiratory stimulus, leading to hypoventilation and carbon dioxide retention (hypercapnia).

- **Dry mucous membranes**: Dry oxygen can irritate the upper airways. Humidifiers can help prevent this discomfort.

- **Fire hazard**: Oxygen promotes combustion. It's essential to keep away from sources of heat or flame, to prohibit smoking in the vicinity, and to follow safety instructions.

- **Barotrauma**: At high pressures, particularly during assisted ventilation, there's a risk of lung damage.

Clinical monitoring of the patient is paramount. It includes assessment of respiratory rate, heart rate, skin coloration, and above all measurement of oxygen saturation (SpO$_2$) using a pulse oximeter. Arterial blood gases can be taken for a more precise analysis of oxygenation and ventilation.

The role of healthcare professionals

Caregivers play a crucial role in the safe and effective use of oxygen therapy:

- **Initial assessment**: Identify signs of hypoxia, understand the patient's specific needs and choose the appropriate mode of administration.

- **Device installation**: Ensure that the equipment is correctly installed, functional and suitable for the patient.

- **Patient education**: Explain the importance of oxygen therapy, how to use the device at home if necessary, and the precautions to be taken.

- **Continuous monitoring**: Observe clinical signs, check oxygen saturation, adjust flow rate according to medical prescriptions and patient's progress.

- **Care coordination**: Collaborate with the multidisciplinary team, report abnormalities, participate in decisions concerning treatment adaptation.

Home oxygen therapy

For patients requiring prolonged oxygen therapy, treatment can be continued at home. This requires specific organization:

- **Equipment** : Oxygen concentrators are the most commonly used devices in the home. They extract oxygen from ambient air and concentrate it for the patient.

- **Training**: Patients and their relatives must be trained in device use, safety precautions and basic maintenance.

- **Regular follow-up**: Home visits by healthcare professionals ensure the proper use of oxygen therapy and the patient's state of health.

- **Lifestyle adaptation**: Adjustments may be needed to integrate oxygen therapy into daily life, while maintaining appropriate physical activity and social participation.

Benefits of oxygen therapy

When used appropriately, oxygen therapy has many benefits:

- **Improved organ function**: By correcting hypoxemia, it enables organs to function optimally.

- **Symptomatic relief**: Reduced dyspnea, increased exercise tolerance, improved sleep.

- **Improved quality of life**: Patients can regain a degree of autonomy and participate more fully in daily activities.

- **Reduced mortality**: In patients with severe COPD and chronic hypoxemia, long-term oxygen therapy has been shown to increase survival.

Ethical and relational considerations

Oxygen therapy, as a potentially invasive and restrictive treatment, raises ethical questions:

- **Informed consent**: The patient must be informed of the benefits, risks and alternatives, and agree to the treatment.

- **Respect for autonomy**: Patient preferences and values must be taken into account in treatment decisions.

- **Empathetic communication**: Caregivers must listen to patients' concerns, answer their questions and support them in their care.

Musculoskeletal disorders

- Osteoarthritis and rheumatism: pain management

Osteoarthritis and rheumatism represent a group of pathologies affecting joints, bones, muscles and connective tissues. These conditions, often chronic, are responsible for persistent pain, stiffness and functional limitations that considerably affect patients' quality of life. Managing the pain associated with osteoarthritis and rheumatism is a major medical challenge, requiring a comprehensive, personalized approach to relieve symptoms, improve mobility and preserve the autonomy of sufferers.

Osteoarthritis, the most common form of joint disease, is a progressive degeneration of the cartilage that covers the bony ends of joints. This wear leads to increased friction between the bones, causing pain, inflammation and the formation of bony outgrowths called osteophytes. The joints most frequently affected are the knees, hips, hands and spine. Rheumatism encompasses a broad spectrum of inflammatory diseases, including rheumatoid arthritis, systemic lupus erythematosus and ankylosing spondylitis. These conditions are characterized by chronic inflammation of the joints and surrounding tissues, often of autoimmune origin, leading to diffuse joint pain, deformity and impaired joint function.

The pain associated with osteoarthritis and rheumatism is complex and multidimensional. It results from nociceptive, inflammatory and neuropathic mechanisms, involving not only joint structures but also nerve pathways and the central nervous system. This chronic pain can have significant physical, psychological and social repercussions, such as fatigue, depression, anxiety and social isolation.

Pain management in these conditions relies on a multimodal approach, combining pharmacological and non-pharmacological interventions, tailored to the patient's needs and preferences. The aim is to reduce pain, improve joint function, prevent deformity and maintain a satisfactory quality of life.

Pharmacologically speaking, analgesics are the mainstay of symptomatic treatment. Paracetamol is often used as a first-line treatment, as it is well-tolerated and effective for mild to moderate pain. Non-steroidal anti-inflammatory drugs (NSAIDs), such as ibuprofen or naproxen, are effective in reducing inflammation and pain, but their use must be cautious due to potential side effects on the digestive, renal and cardiovascular systems. In patients with contraindications to NSAIDs, alternatives such as selective COX-2 inhibitors may be considered.

In cases of severe pain or pain resistant to first-line treatments, weak opioids such as tramadol or codeine can be prescribed with careful monitoring to avoid the risk of dependence or adverse effects. Intra-articular corticosteroid infiltrations are an option for temporarily relieving pain and inflammation in affected joints, particularly when systemic treatments are insufficient or contraindicated.

Disease-modifying therapies, particularly for inflammatory rheumatism, aim to modify disease progression and prevent joint damage. Disease-modifying antirheumatic drugs (DMARDs), such as methotrexate, sulfasalazine or biotherapies targeting pro-inflammatory cytokines, are essential for controlling disease activity and reducing lesion progression.

In addition to drugs, non-pharmacological approaches play a crucial role in managing pain and improving joint function. Patient education is essential to enable patients to understand their disease, actively participate in its management and adopt health-promoting behaviours. Physiotherapy is essential to maintain or restore joint mobility, strengthen muscles, improve balance and prevent deformity. Appropriate exercises, performed under professional supervision, help reduce pain and improve functional capacity.

Occupational therapy helps patients to adapt their daily activities and environment, and to use technical aids to preserve their independence and reduce stress on painful joints. Thermotherapy techniques, such as the application of heat or cold, can provide symptomatic relief by reducing local pain and inflammation.

Complementary therapies, such as acupuncture, relaxation, meditation or yoga, can also be beneficial in reducing stress, improving general well-being and modulating pain perception. A psychosocial approach is important to address the emotional and relational aspects of chronic pain. Psychological support or cognitive-behavioural therapy can help patients to develop strategies for managing pain and associated anxiety or depression.

Nutritional management can also influence pain management in osteoarthritis and rheumatism. A balanced diet, rich in antioxidants, omega-3 fatty acids and essential nutrients, helps reduce systemic inflammation. Weight loss in overweight or obese patients is particularly beneficial in reducing the mechanical load on weight-bearing joints, such as knees and hips, and in alleviating pain.

Orthopedic surgery is considered when conservative treatments are insufficient, and pain or disability significantly impair quality of life. Surgical interventions, such as arthroplasty (joint replacement), can restore joint function, reduce pain and improve mobility. However, these procedures carry risks and require a careful assessment of the benefits and drawbacks for each individual patient.

Care coordination is essential to ensure comprehensive, coherent care. Healthcare professionals, including GPs, rheumatologists, physiotherapists, occupational therapists, nurses and psychologists, need to work closely together to develop a personalized care plan tailored to the patient's specific needs.

It's important to stress that pain management in osteoarthritis and rheumatism is an ongoing process, requiring regular reassessment of treatments and interventions. Active listening to patients, taking into account their preferences and personal goals, are key elements in optimizing the effectiveness of management and encouraging adherence to treatment.

- Osteoporosis: preventing fractures

Osteoporosis is a bone disease characterized by a reduction in the density and quality of bones, making them fragile and prone to fracture. It is often referred to as a "silent disease", as it progresses without apparent symptoms until a fracture occurs. Preventing osteoporosis-related fractures is a major public health issue, particularly for the elderly, as these fractures can have serious consequences for mobility, independence and quality of life.

Understanding osteoporosis

With age, natural bone remodeling becomes unbalanced: bone resorption (destruction of bone tissue) exceeds bone formation. This process leads to a progressive loss of bone mass.

Osteoporosis is characterized by increased porosity of bone tissue, reducing its mechanical strength and increasing the risk of fractures, even following minor trauma.

Risk factors

Several factors contribute to the development of osteoporosis:

- **Age**: Risk increases with age, especially after 50.
- **Gender**: Women are more affected, especially after the menopause, due to the drop in estrogen, which plays a protective role in bone mass.
- **Family history**: Genetic predisposition may increase risk.
- **Morphology**: People of short stature or low weight are at increased risk.
- **Nutritional deficiencies**: Inadequate calcium and vitamin D intake affects bone health.
- **Sedentary lifestyle**: Lack of physical activity reduces the stimulation needed to maintain bone density.
- **Smoking and alcohol**: Smoking and excessive alcohol consumption are detrimental to bone health.
- **Certain diseases and medications**: Endocrine or digestive disorders, or prolonged use of corticosteroids, can favour osteoporosis.

Fracture prevention

Preventing osteoporosis-related fractures is based on a number of complementary approaches designed to strengthen bones and reduce the risk of falls.

1. **A balanced diet rich in essential nutrients**

    - **Calcium**: Key mineral for bone formation and maintenance. Daily requirements vary according to age, but adults generally need between 1,000 and 1,200 mg of calcium per day. Food sources include dairy products (milk, yoghurt, cheese),

- green leafy vegetables (broccoli, kale), almonds and fish with edible bones such as sardines.
  - **Vitamin D**: Facilitates the body's absorption of calcium. Vitamin D is synthesized by the skin under the effect of sunlight, and is also found in certain foods such as oily fish (salmon, mackerel), liver and eggs. Supplementation may be necessary, especially in winter or for the elderly whose skin synthesis is reduced.
  - **Protein**: Essential for bone health, but must be consumed in adequate quantities. Sources include meat, fish, legumes and dairy products.
  - **Other nutrients**: Magnesium, phosphorus, zinc and vitamins K and C also play a role in bone health.

2. **Regular physical activity**

   - **Weight-bearing exercise**: Activities that challenge the bones against gravity, such as walking, dancing and jogging, help build bone density.
   - **Muscle-strengthening exercises**: Training with weights or elastic bands improves muscle strength, supporting bones and reducing the risk of falls.
   - **Balance and coordination exercises**: Tai chi, yoga or gentle gymnastics help prevent falls by improving stability and proprioception.

3. **Healthy lifestyle**

   - **Smoking cessation**: Smoking accelerates bone loss and increases the risk of fractures.
   - **Limiting alcohol**: Excessive alcohol consumption is detrimental to bone formation and increases the risk of falls.

- **Stress management**: High levels of stress can affect bone health. Relaxation techniques and good sleep hygiene are beneficial.

4. **Screening and monitoring**

    - **Fracture risk assessment**: Tools such as the FRAX score can be used to estimate 10-year fracture risk based on a number of clinical factors.
    - **Bone densitometry**: This examination measures bone mineral density (BMD) and helps diagnose osteoporosis. It is recommended for women over 65 and men over 70, or earlier in the presence of risk factors.
    - **Regular medical follow-up**: to monitor bone density and adapt preventive or therapeutic measures.

5. **Drug treatments**

    When preventive measures are not sufficient, or in cases of proven osteoporosis, treatments may be prescribed:

    - **Bisphosphonates**: Reduce bone resorption by inhibiting osteoclast activity. Reduces the risk of vertebral and non-vertebral fractures.
    - **Selective estrogen receptor modulators (SERMs)**: act like estrogen on bones, without the side effects on breasts or uterus.
    - **Denosumab**: A monoclonal antibody that inhibits osteoclast formation and activity.
    - **Hormonal therapies**: Hormone replacement therapy (HRT) may be considered for post-menopausal women, but must be weighed up against the risks and benefits.
    - **Bone anabolics**: like teriparatide, promote bone formation.

6. These treatments require medical follow-up to monitor efficacy and possible side effects.

7. **Preventing falls**
   Osteoporotic fractures often result from falls, particularly in the elderly. Preventing falls is therefore essential:
   - **Home improvements**: Eliminate obstacles, secure carpets, install grab bars in bathrooms, ensure good lighting.
   - **Correcting visual problems**: Regular eye examinations to correct eyesight.
   - **Suitable footwear**: Wear non-slip, well-fitting shoes.
   - **Medication evaluation** : Some medications can cause dizziness or affect balance. A review of treatments with the doctor may be necessary.
   - **Balance training programs**: Participate in specific workshops to improve stability and reduce the risk of falling.

8. **Education and awareness**
   - **Disease information**: Understanding osteoporosis helps patients adhere to preventive measures.
   - **Support groups**: Join associations or patient groups to share experiences and advice.

- Mobilization assistance with respect for limitations

Patient mobilization is an essential component of nursing care and support for people in temporary or permanent dependency situations. It aims to maintain or improve physical mobility, prevent complications associated with immobility and promote autonomy. However, each patient has specific abilities and limitations that must be respected to ensure safe and caring care. This article explores the fundamental principles of assisted mobilization, taking into account individual limitations, with an emphasis on appropriate techniques, the role of caregivers and the importance of a person-centered approach.

Understanding the patient's limitations

Before undertaking any mobilization action, it is essential to understand the patient's limitations, whether physical, cognitive or emotional. These limitations may be due to a variety of factors:

1. **Physical limitations** :

    - **Muscular weakness**: due to illness, surgery or prolonged immobilization.
    - **Pain**: Present during movement, it can impair mobility.
    - **Balance disorders**: Increased risk of falls during mobilization.
    - **Joint limitations**: stiffness, contractures or restrictions of movement due to pathologies such as osteoarthritis.
    - **Partial or complete paralysis**: the result of a stroke or spinal cord injury.

2. **Cognitive limitations** :

    - **Mental confusion**: Difficulty understanding instructions or cooperating.
    - **Memory problems**: forget safety instructions.
    - **Disorientation**: Risk of inappropriate or dangerous movements.

3. **Emotional and psychological limitations** :

    - **Anxiety or fear**: Fear of pain, falling or the unknown.

- **Lack of motivation**: Depression or apathy reducing commitment to mobilization.
- **Refusal to cooperate**: Opposition to care for various reasons.

Basic principles for respectful mobilization

1. **Initial assessment** :

   - **Observation**: Note posture, spontaneous movements, facial expressions indicating pain.
   - **Communication**: Discuss with patients to understand their feelings, fears and expectations.
   - **Consulting medical records**: Knowing the history, diagnoses, prescriptions and recommendations of healthcare professionals.

2. **Mobilization planning** :

   - **Set realistic goals**: Adapt activities to the patient's current abilities.
   - **Choose appropriate techniques**: Use transfer or mobilization methods adapted to identified limitations.
   - **Preparing the environment**: Ensure a safe, uncluttered area equipped with the necessary technical aids.

3. **Effective communication** :

   - **Clear explanation**: Inform the patient of the mobilization procedure, the steps involved and what is expected of him or her.
   - **Active listening**: Encourage patients to express their concerns or discomfort.
   - **Positive reinforcement**: Valorize the patient's efforts, however small, to boost confidence and motivation.

4. **Respecting the patient's rhythm**:

    - **Patience**: Allow the patient time to carry out the movements, without rushing them.
    - **Adaptation**: Modify the plan if the patient encounters unexpected difficulties.
    - **Rest**: Take breaks if necessary to avoid excessive fatigue.

5. **Safety first**:

    - **Use of technical aids**: wheelchairs, walkers, bed rails, transfer belts.
    - **Correct positioning**: Ensure correct posture to prevent injury to patient and caregiver.
    - **Appropriate assistance**: Ask a colleague for help if mobilization requires several people.

Adapted mobilization techniques

1. **Bed-chair transfer**:

    - **Preparation**: Check that the bed and chair brakes are activated.
    - **Positioning**: Help the patient to sit on the edge of the bed, feet flat on the floor.
    - **Use of a transfer belt**: Facilitate the patient's grip and support.
    - **Accompanying movement**: Encourage patients to participate by pushing on their legs if possible.

2. **Walking aids**:

    - **Balance assessment**: Ensure that the patient can stand safely.
    - **Using a walker or cane**: Offer extra support.

- **Caregiver positioning**: Stand slightly back and to the side, ready to support in case of imbalance.

3. **Changes of position in bed** :

    - **Pressure sore prevention**: Regularly change the patient's position to avoid prolonged pressure points.
    - **Turning techniques**: Use a sliding sheet or undersheet to facilitate movement.
    - **Respecting pain**: avoid sudden movements, be attentive to the patient's reactions.

4. **Passive mobilization**:

    - **For patients unable to move independently**: The caregiver performs movements to maintain joint mobility.
    - **Gentle, gradual amplitude**: Do not force joints beyond the point of resistance or pain.
    - **Observing reactions**: Watch for signs of pain or fatigue.

The caregiver's role in respecting limitations

1. **Technical skills** :

    - **Ongoing training**: Keep abreast of new mobilization techniques and safety protocols.
    - **Gesture control** : Ensure precise execution to avoid injury.

2. **Empathy and respect** :

    - **Recognition of individuality**: Every patient is unique, with his or her own needs and preferences.

- **Confidentiality and dignity**: Respect privacy during mobilizations, especially in the presence of other people.

3. **Interprofessional collaboration** :

    - **Communication with the team**: Share observations and difficulties encountered to adapt the care plan.
    - **Coordination with physiotherapists**: Incorporate recommendations from rehabilitation specialists.

4. **Promoting independence** :

    - **Encouraging participation**: Motivate patients to perform movements they can do on their own.
    - **Education**: Provide advice on independent exercise, where appropriate.

The importance of a suitable environment

1. **Security** :

    - **Obstacle removal**: Make sure the floor is clear of slippery mats and bulky objects.
    - **Adequate lighting**: Facilitate visibility to prevent falls.

2. **Appropriate equipment** :

    - **Adjustable beds**: Enable height adjustment to facilitate transfers.
    - **Grab bars**: Install supports in key areas such as the bathroom.
    - **Technical aids**: Use lifts or transfer boards if necessary.

Patient-centered approach

1. **Taking preferences into account** :
   - **Schedules**: Mobilize patients at times that suit them, respecting their biological rhythms.
   - **Methods**: Adapt techniques according to what is most comfortable for the patient.

2. **Cultural and spiritual respect**:
   - **Sensitivity to beliefs**: Take into account cultural or religious practices that may influence mobilization.
   - **Appropriate language**: Use respectful terms and avoid incomprehensible medical jargon.

3. **Psychological support** :
   - **Managing anxiety**: Use relaxation or distraction techniques to calm the patient.
   - **Building trust**: Establishing a relationship of trust through reliability and benevolence.

Managing difficult situations

1. **Refusal to mobilize** :
   - **Understanding the reasons**: Identify whether the refusal is related to pain, fear or confusion.
   - **Negotiation**: Propose alternatives or postpone mobilization if possible.
   - **Finding solutions**: Involve the care team or loved ones in finding appropriate strategies.

2. **Pain on mobilization** :
   - **Pain assessment**: Use appropriate scales to measure pain intensity.

- **Analgesic treatment**: Administer prescribed medication prior to mobilization.
- **Adapting movements**: Reduce amplitude or modify technique to minimize pain.

Diabetes in the Elderly

- Blood glucose monitoring

Glycemia, the level of glucose in the blood, is an essential biological parameter for the proper functioning of the body. Glucose is the main source of energy for cells, particularly those in the brain and muscles. Regulation of blood glucose levels is therefore crucial to maintaining homeostasis and preventing metabolic complications. Blood glucose monitoring is a fundamental practice, particularly for people with diabetes, to ensure optimal control of their health.

Diabetes is a chronic disease characterized by persistent hyperglycemia due to insufficient insulin production (type 1 diabetes), insulin resistance (type 2 diabetes) or both. Without proper management, diabetes can lead to serious complications such as cardiovascular disease, kidney damage, nerve damage and vision problems. Regular blood glucose monitoring enables patients and healthcare professionals to make informed decisions about treatment, diet and lifestyle.

Understanding blood sugar regulation

Blood glucose levels are regulated by a complex balance between glucose production by the liver, food intake and glucose utilization by cells. Insulin, a hormone secreted by the beta cells of the pancreas, plays a key role in facilitating the entry of glucose into cells, thereby reducing blood glucose levels. Glucagon, produced by the alpha cells of the pancreas, has the opposite effect, stimulating the liver to release glucose when blood glucose levels are low.

In healthy people, this regulatory system maintains blood sugar levels within a normal range, generally between 70 and 110 mg/dL on an empty stomach. However, various factors can disrupt this balance, necessitating increased monitoring.

Why monitor blood sugar levels?

Blood glucose monitoring is essential for several reasons:

1. **Diabetes control**: It enables doses of insulin or other hypoglycemic drugs to be adjusted according to variations in blood sugar levels.

2. **Prevention of hypoglycemia and hyperglycemia**: By identifying abnormalities early on, patients can take steps to correct their blood sugar levels.

3. **Assessment of treatment effectiveness**: This helps determine whether the current treatment plan is effective or needs to be modified.

4. **Understanding the impact of diet and physical activity**: Provides an overview of how meals, exercise and other factors influence blood glucose levels.

5. **Prevention of long-term complications**: Strict glycemic control reduces the risk of microvascular and macrovascular complications.

Blood glucose monitoring methods

Blood glucose monitoring can be carried out in different ways:

1. **Capillary blood glucose**: This is the most common method, involving a small prick on the fingertip to obtain a drop of blood, which is analyzed by a portable glucometer. This method is fast, convenient and can be performed at home.

2. **Venous blood glucose**: Performed in a laboratory, it provides an accurate measure of blood glucose, but is not practical for frequent monitoring.

3. **Continuous glucose monitoring systems (CGM)**: These devices continuously measure interstitial blood glucose levels using a sensor placed under the skin. They provide real-time data and warn of hypo- or hyperglycemia.

4. **Glycated hemoglobin (HbA1c)**: This indicator reflects average blood glucose levels over the past two to three months. Although it does not replace daily monitoring, it is essential for assessing long-term glycemic control.

How to monitor blood sugar levels correctly?

Effective monitoring requires the right technique:

1. **Preparation**: Wash hands with warm water and soap to avoid contamination which could falsify results. Dry hands thoroughly before measuring.

2. **Start measurement**: Insert a test strip into the meter according to the manufacturer's instructions.

3. **Obtaining the blood sample**: Use a sterile lancet to prick the side of the fingertip (less painful than the center). Light pressure may help to obtain a sufficient drop of blood.

4. **Blood application**: Touch the drop of blood to the strip, making sure there is enough for an accurate reading.

5. **Reading the result**: Wait for the meter to display the blood glucose level, usually within a few seconds. Note the result, the time and the circumstances (before or after a meal, after exercise, etc.).

6. **Waste management**: dispose of used lancets and strips in a sharps container to prevent injury and infection.

Interpretation of results

Understanding blood glucose values is essential for taking appropriate action:

- **Normal fasting blood glucose**: between 70 and 110 mg/dL.
- **Postprandial blood glucose (2 hours after a meal)**: below 140 mg/dL for non-diabetics. For diabetics, targets may vary according to medical recommendations.

Values below 70 mg/dL indicate hypoglycemia, requiring immediate action, such as the consumption of fast carbohydrates. Values above recommended targets may require adjustment of treatment or modifications to diet and physical activity.

Monitoring frequency

The frequency of monitoring depends on the type of diabetes, treatment and medical recommendations:

- **Type 1 diabetes**: frequent monitoring, usually before meals, at bedtime and sometimes at night.
- **Type 2 diabetes on insulin**: Monitoring before meals and at bedtime.
- **Type 2 diabetes on oral medication**: The frequency may be lower, but regular monitoring is recommended to assess treatment efficacy.
- **Special situations**: In the event of illness, change of treatment, travel, or symptoms of hypo- or hyperglycemia, increased monitoring is required.

Technological advances in blood glucose monitoring

Technologies have considerably improved blood glucose monitoring:

1. **Continuous glucose monitoring (CGM) systems**: provide a complete picture of blood glucose variations, helping to identify trends and prevent hypo- or hyperglycemic episodes.

2. **Insulin pumps coupled with CGMs**: They can automatically adjust insulin delivery according to blood glucose readings, improving diabetes control.

3. **Mobile applications and software**: These can be used to monitor blood glucose levels, diet, physical activity and other parameters, making it easier to manage diabetes.

4. **Non-injection glucose meters**: Research is underway to develop non-invasive devices that measure blood glucose levels using optical methods or electromagnetic interference.

Challenges and considerations

Despite the benefits, blood glucose monitoring can present challenges:

- **Pain and discomfort**: Repeated injections can be painful and discouraging.

- **Cost**: Strips, lancets and devices may represent a financial burden.

- **Adherence**: The daily monitoring routine can be restrictive, leading to reduced compliance.

- **Accuracy of measurements**: Operating errors or equipment faults can lead to inaccurate readings.

The role of healthcare professionals

Healthcare professionals play a crucial role in monitoring blood sugar levels:

- **Therapeutic education**: Train patients in correct measurement technique, interpretation of results and decision-making.

- **Personalizing the care plan**: Adapt glycemic targets and monitoring frequency to individual needs.

- **Psychological support**: Helping patients overcome the emotional obstacles associated with managing diabetes.

- **Regular monitoring**: assess glycemic control, adjust treatments and prevent complications.

- Signs of hypo- and hyperglycemia

Regulation of blood sugar levels is essential for the body to function properly. Glucose is the main source of energy for cells, particularly those in the brain. A disturbance in blood sugar levels, whether too low (hypoglycemia) or too high (hyperglycemia), can have serious consequences for health. So it's crucial to recognize the warning signs of these imbalances so you can act quickly to prevent complications.

Understanding blood sugar and its regulation

The body maintains blood sugar levels within a narrow range thanks to the action of several hormones, mainly insulin and glucagon, produced by the pancreas. Insulin enables cells to absorb glucose from the blood, thereby lowering blood sugar levels, while glucagon stimulates the liver to release glucose when blood sugar levels are too low. In people with diabetes, this mechanism is altered, which can lead to episodes of hypoglycemia or hyperglycemia.

Hypoglycemia

Definition and causes

Hypoglycemia occurs when blood glucose levels fall below 70 mg/dL (3.9 mmol/L). It is common in diabetics treated with insulin or certain hypoglycemic drugs. Common causes include an excessive dose of insulin, a delayed or forgotten meal, intense physical activity without adjustment of carbohydrate intake, or fasting alcohol consumption.

Signs and symptoms of hypoglycemia

The manifestations of hypoglycemia result from the response of the autonomic nervous system and the lack of glucose available to the brain.

1. **Early signs (adrenergic response)** :

    - **Excessive sweating**: cold, clammy sweat, especially on the forehead and nape of the neck.
    - **Tremors** : Hand tremors, sometimes generalized.
    - **Palpitations**: sensation of rapid or irregular heartbeat.
    - **Anxiety or nervousness**: unexplained feelings of anxiety.
    - **Sudden hunger**: Urgent need to eat, especially sweet foods.

2. **Neuroglycopenic signs (lack of glucose in the brain)** :

    - **Weakness or fatigue**: Sudden feeling of lassitude.
    - Difficulty **concentrating**, mental confusion.

- **Visual disturbances**: blurred or double vision.
- **Headaches**: Mild to severe headaches.
- **Speech disorders**: difficulty speaking clearly, stuttering.
- **Mood swings**: irritability, aggressiveness, depression.

3. **Severe signs** :

    - **Loss of coordination**: Difficulty walking or performing precise movements.
    - **Convulsions**: epileptiform seizures in cases of profound hypoglycemia.
    - **Loss of consciousness**: fainting, hypoglycemic coma if untreated.

Consequences if left untreated

Severe, uncorrected hypoglycemia can lead to permanent brain damage or even death. It is therefore vital to intervene rapidly by administering sugar (orally if the patient is conscious, or by injection of glucagon or intravenous glucose in a medical setting).

Hyperglycemia

Definition and causes

Hyperglycemia is characterized by a rise in blood glucose above 126 mg/dL (7 mmol/L) fasting or 200 mg/dL (11.1 mmol/L) two hours after a meal. It is common among diabetics, particularly if treatment is inadequate or poorly adapted. Causes include excessive carbohydrate intake, insufficient insulin or medication, stress, infection or reduced physical activity.

Signs and symptoms of hyperglycemia

The symptoms of hyperglycemia are often insidious and can go unnoticed, especially in the early stages.

1. **Classic signs**:

   - **Excessive thirst (polydipsia)**: The need to drink frequently and in large quantities.
   - **Frequent urination (polyuria)**: The need to urinate often, including at night (nocturia).
   - **Fatigue**: Persistent feeling of tiredness, even after rest.
   - **Blurred vision**: difficulty seeing clearly, visual fluctuations.
   - **Involuntary weight loss**: Despite normal or increased appetite.
   - **Increased appetite (polyphagia)**: constant feeling of hunger.

2. **Skin signs** :

   - **Dry skin**: skin dehydration, itching.
   - **Recurrent infections**: Skin infections, candidiasis, urinary tract infections.

3. **Severe signs (in cases of prolonged or very high hyperglycemia)** :

   - **Sleepiness**: Difficulty staying awake, lethargy.
   - **Mental confusion**: disorientation, disturbed consciousness.
   - **Nausea and vomiting**: Particularly in diabetic ketoacidosis.
   - **Abdominal pain**: associated with the accumulation of ketone bodies.
   - **Kussmaul breathing**: deep, rapid breathing to compensate for acidosis.

- **Fruity breath**: Acetone odor due to ketone bodies.

Consequences if left untreated

Severe hyperglycemia can lead to serious acute complications:

- **Diabetic ketoacidosis**: Especially in patients with type 1 diabetes, characterized by an accumulation of ketone bodies, causing metabolic acidosis.
- **Hyperglycemic hyperosmolar syndrome**: More common in elderly patients with type 2 diabetes, leading to severe dehydration and altered consciousness.

These conditions require urgent medical attention to rehydrate the patient, correct electrolyte imbalances and administer insulin.

The importance of early recognition

Early identification of signs of hypo- or hyperglycemia enables prompt action to correct blood sugar levels and avoid complications. Diabetic patients and those around them need to be informed and trained to recognize these signs and know how to react.

What to do in the event of hypoglycemia?

1. **Measure blood glucose**: If possible, to confirm hypoglycemia.
2. **Eat fast carbohydrates**: Take 15 grams of fast-absorbing carbohydrates, such as :
   - 3 sugar cubes.
   - One glass of fruit juice (150 ml).
   - A tablespoon of honey or jam.

3. **Wait 15 minutes**: Then recheck blood glucose.
4. **If symptoms persist**: Take another 15 grams of fast carbohydrates.
5. **Have a snack**: Once blood sugar has been corrected, eat complex carbohydrates to stabilize blood sugar levels.
6. **If unconscious**: Give nothing by mouth. Call emergency services and, if available, administer glucagon by injection.

What to do in case of hyperglycemia?

1. **Measuring blood glucose**: To assess the level of hyperglycemia.
2. **Hydration**: Drink water to prevent dehydration.
3. **Insulin administration**: adjust insulin dose according to medical recommendations.
4. **Avoid strenuous physical effort**: this can aggravate hyperglycemia in the presence of ketone bodies.
5. **Monitor symptoms**: If values remain high, or if signs are severe, consult a doctor or go to the emergency room.

Prevention of hypo- and hyperglycemic episodes

- **Regular monitoring**: Check blood glucose levels frequently to anticipate variations.
- **Compliance with treatment**: Take medication or insulin as prescribed.
- **Balanced diet**: adapt carbohydrate intake according to treatment and activity.
- **Adapted physical activity**: Take part in regular physical activity in line with medical advice.
- **Stress management**: Stress can influence blood sugar levels; relaxation techniques can help.
- **Therapeutic education**: Participate in educational programs to better manage your diabetes.

- Suitable diet

The right diet is essential for maintaining good health, preventing disease and optimizing body functions. It is a personalized diet that takes into account individual nutritional needs, medical conditions, lifestyle, cultural and taste preferences. This approach not only satisfies nutritional requirements, but also promotes general well-being and quality of life.

Fundamentals of an adapted diet

1. **Nutritional balance**

    An appropriate diet must provide a balanced intake of macronutrients (carbohydrates, proteins, lipids) and micronutrients (vitamins, minerals, trace elements). The balance between these elements is crucial for proper metabolic function, growth, tissue repair and energy production.

2. **Personalized**

    Each individual has specific nutritional needs based on age, gender, height, weight, level of physical activity and state of health. An adapted diet takes these factors into account to adjust caloric and nutritional intake.

3. **Food quality**

    The quality of the food we eat has a major influence on our health. It's important to choose fresh, unprocessed foods that are rich in nutrients and low in harmful substances. Fruits, vegetables, whole grains, lean proteins and healthy fats form the basis of a healthy diet.

4. **Respect for cultural and personal preferences**

    A diet must be compatible with the individual's cultural traditions, religious beliefs and taste preferences. This facilitates long-term adherence to the diet and contributes to the pleasure of eating.

5. **Adapting to medical conditions**
    In the presence of certain medical conditions such as diabetes, hypertension, food allergies or kidney disease, it is necessary to adapt the diet to manage the disease and prevent complications.

Key components of an adapted diet

1. **Carbohydrates**
    Carbohydrates are the body's main source of energy. We recommend giving preference to the complex carbohydrates found in whole grains, legumes and certain vegetables. These foods provide long-lasting energy and are rich in fiber, which promotes satiety and digestive health.

2. **Proteins**
    Proteins are essential for tissue construction and repair, enzyme and hormone production. Protein sources can be animal-based (lean meat, poultry, fish, eggs, dairy products) or plant-based (legumes, nuts, seeds, soy). It is beneficial to vary sources to obtain a complete amino acid profile.

3. **Fats**
    Fats are essential for the absorption of fat-soluble vitamins, the production of hormones and the proper functioning of the nervous system. It's best to opt for the unsaturated fats found in vegetable oils, avocados, nuts and omega-3-rich fatty fish, while limiting saturated and trans fats.

4. **Vitamins and minerals**
    These micronutrients are essential for many biological functions. A varied diet rich in colorful fruits and vegetables ensures an adequate supply of essential vitamins and minerals.

5. **Hydration**
Water is vital for transporting nutrients, regulating body temperature and eliminating waste. It's important to drink enough water throughout the day, adjusting intake according to physical activity and climatic conditions.

Adapting the plan to specific conditions

1. **Diabetes**
For diabetics, controlling blood sugar levels is essential. A suitable diet includes :

   - **Carbohydrate control**: balanced distribution of complex carbohydrates with low glycemic index to avoid glycemic peaks.
   - **Dietary fiber**: Increase fiber intake to slow glucose absorption.
   - **Healthy fats**: Choose unsaturated fats to protect cardiovascular health.

2. **Hypertension**
Hypertension management involves :

   - **Sodium reduction**: Limit salt intake by avoiding processed foods and cooking with herbs and spices.
   - **Increase potassium**: Eat potassium-rich foods such as bananas, spinach and potatoes to help regulate blood pressure.
   - **DASH diet**: Adoption of the Dietary Approaches to Stop Hypertension diet, rich in fruits, vegetables, low-fat dairy products and whole grains.

3. **Hypercholesterolemia**
To lower cholesterol levels:

- **Limit saturated fats**: Reduce fatty meats, full-fat dairy products and fried foods.
- **Soluble fiber**: Eat oats, legumes and fruit to reduce cholesterol absorption.
- **Plant sterols**: Inclusion of sterol-enriched foods to lower LDL cholesterol.

4. **Food allergies and intolerances**

   It's crucial to identify and eliminate trigger foods, while taking care to compensate for missing nutrients. For example:

   - **Lactose intolerance**: Replace dairy products with lactose-free or calcium-enriched alternatives.
   - **Gluten allergy**: Use gluten-free cereals such as rice, corn or quinoa.

5. **Kidney disease**

   A specific diet can help reduce the burden on the kidneys:

   - **Protein restriction**: Limiting protein intake to slow the progression of renal failure.
   - **Sodium, potassium and phosphorus control**: adjusting intakes to prevent electrolyte imbalances.

Tips for setting up a suitable diet

1. **Consultation with a professional**

   Calling on the services of a dietician or nutritionist can help you develop a personalized eating plan that takes into account your specific needs and health objectives.

2. **Meal planning**

   Planning meals in advance helps maintain a balanced diet and avoid less healthy impulsive choices.

3. **Reading labels**
   Learning to decipher the nutritional information on packaging enables you to make informed choices, limiting added sugars, saturated fats and sodium.

4. **Cooking at home**
   Preparing your own meals gives you greater control over the ingredients you use and the cooking methods you use, promoting healthier eating.

5. **Adopting reasonable portion sizes**
   Understanding and respecting recommended portion sizes helps avoid caloric excess and maintain a healthy weight.

6. **Gradual integration of changes**
   Gradual introduction of new eating habits promotes lasting adaptation, rather than an abrupt, restrictive approach.

Benefits of an adapted diet

- **Improved general health**: Reduced risk of chronic diseases such as cardiovascular disease, diabetes and certain cancers.

- **Weight management**: Maintain a healthy body weight by balancing energy intake and expenditure.

- **Mental well-being**: Good nutrition has a positive influence on mood, cognition and energy levels.

- **Longevity**: A healthy diet helps extend healthy life expectancy.

Chapter 5

Emergency situations and first aid procedures

Recognizing emergency signs

- Respiratory distress

Respiratory distress is a critical medical situation characterized by acute insufficiency of respiratory function, resulting in an inability to ensure adequate gas exchange between ambient air and blood. This condition compromises the supply of oxygen to tissues and the elimination of carbon dioxide, which can rapidly become life-threatening. Rapid recognition of the signs of respiratory distress and immediate medical intervention are essential to prevent serious, even fatal, complications.

Pathophysiology of respiratory distress

The main function of the respiratory system is to oxygenate the blood and eliminate the carbon dioxide produced by cellular metabolism. Respiratory distress occurs when this process is disrupted, whether by airway obstruction, altered pulmonary mechanics, respiratory muscle weakness or dysregulation of neurological control of breathing.

Several mechanisms may be at the root of this disturbance:

1. **Airway obstruction**: A foreign body, inflammatory edema, severe asthma attack or allergic reaction can partially or totally obstruct the airway, preventing the passage of air.

2. **Impaired alveolar-capillary diffusion**: Diseases such as pneumonia, pulmonary edema or acute respiratory distress syndrome (ARDS) affect the alveoli, reducing the efficiency of gas exchange.

3. **Ventilatory pump dysfunction**: Weak or paralyzed respiratory muscles, as in neuromuscular diseases (myasthenia gravis, Guillain-Barré syndrome), prevent adequate ventilation.

4. **Depression of the respiratory center**: Substances such as opioids, sedatives or brain damage can inhibit neurological control of breathing.

Signs and symptoms of respiratory distress

Early recognition of the signs of respiratory distress is crucial for effective management. Clinical manifestations include:

- **Dyspnea**: Subjective sensation of difficulty in breathing, often described as shortness of breath or chest tightness.

- **Tachypnea**: Acceleration of respiratory rate to compensate for lack of oxygen.

- **Use of accessory muscles**: Engage neck, shoulder and abdominal muscles to facilitate breathing.

- **Nasal flaring**: pronounced movement of the nostrils with each inspiration, especially in children.

- **Intercostal and suprasternal pulling**: Visible indentation of the spaces between the ribs or above the sternum during inspiration.

- **Cyanosis**: Bluish discoloration of lips, nails or skin, indicating severe hypoxemia.

- **Agitation or confusion**: Cerebral hypoxia can cause mental state disorders.

- **Cold sweat**: excessive perspiration linked to respiratory stress.

- **Tachycardia**: Elevated heart rate in response to hypoxemia.

- **Auscultatory silence**: Absence of respiratory sounds on auscultation, a sign of pulmonary obstruction or collapse.

Causes of respiratory distress

Many conditions can lead to respiratory distress:

1. **Acute respiratory infections** :
    - *Pneumonia*: Infection of the pulmonary alveoli by bacteria, viruses or fungi.
    - *Bronchiolitis*: Inflammation of the bronchioles, common in infants.
    - *Epiglottitis*: Inflammation of the epiglottis that can obstruct the upper airway.

2. **Obstructive airway diseases** :
    - *Acute severe asthma*: severe exacerbation of asthma not controlled by usual treatments.
    - *Decompensated COPD*: Sudden worsening of chronic obstructive pulmonary disease.

3. **Thoracic trauma** :
    - *Pneumothorax*: Accumulation of air in the pleural cavity, compressing the lung.
    - *Hemothorax*: Presence of blood in the pleural cavity.

4. **Pulmonary embolism** :
    - Obstruction of the pulmonary arteries by a blood clot, reducing pulmonary perfusion.

5. **Cardiogenic pulmonary edema** :

    ○ Accumulation of fluid in the alveoli due to heart failure.

6. **Severe allergic reactions** :

    ○ *Anaphylaxis*: Intense immune reaction causing airway edema and generalized vasodilation.

7. **Poisoning** :

    ○ *Carbon monoxide*: Odorless gas that binds to hemoglobin, preventing oxygen transport.
    ○ *Drug overdose*: respiratory depression induced by substances such as opioids.

8. **Neuromuscular diseases** :

    ○ Weakening of respiratory muscles compromising ventilation, as in amyotrophic lateral sclerosis.

Diagnosis of respiratory distress

Diagnosis is based on rapid clinical evaluation and additional tests:

1. **Anamnesis**:

    ○ Questioning about symptoms, medical history, recent exposures (allergens, toxins), current treatments.

2. **Physical examination** :

    ○ Observation of vital signs: respiratory rate, heart rate, blood pressure, oxygen saturation.

- Pulmonary auscultation: look for abnormal noises such as sibilants (wheezing), rales or crackles.

3. **Pulse oximetry** :

    - Non-invasive measurement of oxygen saturation (SpO_2) to assess hypoxemia.

4. **Arterial blood gas** :

    - Precise analysis of oxygenation, ventilation ($PaCO_2$) and acid-base balance.

5. **Chest X-ray**:

    - Visualization of lung structures to detect abnormalities such as pneumothorax, pneumonia or pulmonary edema.

6. **Electrocardiogram (ECG)** :

    - Detection of cardiac anomalies that may contribute to respiratory distress.

7. **Blood biology** :

    - Blood count, inflammatory markers, D-dimer in case of suspected pulmonary embolism.

8. **Advanced imaging** :

    - Chest CT scan for a detailed assessment of the lungs and surrounding structures.

Management of respiratory distress

Respiratory distress is a medical emergency requiring immediate intervention:

1. **Ensuring airway patency**:
   - Position the patient in a semi-seated position to facilitate breathing.
   - Remove any obstructions (secretions, foreign bodies) from the respiratory tract.

2. **Oxygen therapy** :
   - Administration of high-flow oxygen via a high-concentration mask to correct hypoxemia.

3. **Assisted ventilation** :
   - Non-invasive ventilation (NIV) with continuous positive airway pressure (CPAP) or bi-level positive airway pressure (BiPAP).
   - Tracheal intubation and mechanical ventilation if NIV is insufficient or contraindicated.

4. **Specific treatment of the cause** :
   - *Asthma or COPD*: Administration of nebulized bronchodilators (salbutamol), systemic corticosteroids.
   - *Pulmonary edema*: diuretics to eliminate excess fluid, vasodilators to reduce cardiac preload.
   - *Pulmonary embolism*: anticoagulation with heparin, thrombolysis if necessary.
   - *Infections* : Appropriate antibiotic therapy for bacterial pneumonia.
   - *Anaphylaxis*: Intramuscular injection of adrenaline, antihistamines, corticosteroids.

5. **Continuous monitoring** :
   - Monitor vital signs, oxygen saturation, heart rate.

- Regular blood gas tests to assess ventilation efficiency.

6. **Transfer to a specialized facility** :
   - Admission to intensive care or resuscitation unit for advanced management.

Preventing respiratory distress

1. **Chronic disease management** :
   - Regular medical follow-up for patients with asthma, COPD or heart failure.
   - Therapeutic education to improve treatment compliance and recognize warning signs.

2. **Vaccinations** :
   - Annual influenza vaccination and pneumococcal vaccination to reduce the risk of serious respiratory infections.

3. **Avoidance of triggers**:
   - Avoid exposure to known allergens, air pollutants and active or passive smoking.

4. **Promoting a healthy lifestyle**:
   - Adopting a balanced diet and regular exercise.

5. **Training for healthcare professionals** :
   - Raising awareness of early recognition of signs of respiratory distress and emergency response protocols.

Psychological impact and patient support

Respiratory distress can be a traumatic experience for the patient, generating anxiety, fear or post-traumatic stress. It is important to :

- **Providing psychological support**: listening, explaining procedures, reassuring patients about their care.

- **Involve the family**: Keep relatives informed, involve them in care if possible to reinforce support.

- **Rehabilitation planning**: After the acute phase, consider respiratory rehabilitation to improve lung function.

- Cardiorespiratory arrest

Cardiorespiratory arrest is an extreme medical emergency characterized by the sudden and simultaneous cessation of cardiac and respiratory functions. This condition rapidly leads to oxygen deprivation in the body, resulting in irreversible damage to vital organs, particularly the brain, if no intervention is carried out within minutes. Immediate and appropriate management of cardiorespiratory arrest is crucial to increase the chances of survival and limit neurological sequelae.

Pathophysiology of cardiopulmonary arrest

The heart and lungs work in close synergy to ensure oxygenation of tissues. The heart pumps oxygenated blood to the organs, while the lungs enrich the blood with oxygen and eliminate carbon dioxide. Cardiorespiratory arrest results from the interruption of these essential functions. The causes may be multiple, but the mechanisms generally lead to acute circulatory failure, preventing the supply of oxygen to the cells.

Causes of cardiorespiratory arrest

1. **Cardiac causes** :

   - **Myocardial infarction**: occlusion of a coronary artery leads to necrosis of heart tissue, which can cause lethal arrhythmias such as ventricular fibrillation.
   - **Cardiac arrhythmias**: rhythm disorders such as ventricular tachycardia or extreme bradycardia disrupt the heart's ability to pump efficiently.
   - **Cardiomyopathies**: Diseases of the heart muscle that weaken the heart's contractile function.

2. **Respiratory causes** :

   - **Airway obstruction**: Choking on a foreign body, angioedema.
   - **Hypoventilation**: drug overdose, opiate intoxication.
   - **Acute pulmonary diseases**: severe pneumonia, massive pulmonary embolism.

3. **Neurological causes** :

   - **Massive stroke**: may disrupt neurological control of breathing and heart rate.
   - **Severe head trauma**: Damage to the brain stem affecting vital regulation centers.

4. **Metabolic and toxic causes** :

   - **Hypoxia**: Lack of oxygen due to asphyxia or carbon monoxide poisoning.
   - **Electrolyte imbalances**: severe hyperkalemia or hypokalemia affecting cardiac activity.

- **Intoxications**: cardiotoxic substances, such as certain drugs or poisons.

5. **External causes** :

    - **Trauma**: massive hemorrhage, electric shock.
    - **Drowning**: Asphyxiation by submersion.

Clinical signs of cardiorespiratory arrest

Rapid recognition of cardiorespiratory arrest is based on the identification of three major signs:

1. **Loss of consciousness**: Patient does not respond to verbal or physical stimuli.

2. **Absence of breathing**: Absence of thoracic movement, no audible or felt breath.

3. **Absence of central pulse**: No palpable carotid or femoral pulses.

Other signs may include cyanosis (bluish coloration of the lips and extremities), mydriasis (dilated pupils) and muscle hypotonia.

Management of cardiorespiratory arrest

Immediate management is crucial, and follows the cardiopulmonary resuscitation (CPR) protocols established by learned societies such as the European Resuscitation Council (ERC) or the American Heart Association (AHA).

1. **Scene safety**: Make sure the environment is safe for both rescuer and patient.

2. **Initial assessment** :

    - Check the patient's reactivity by stimulating him.

- Open the airway by tilting the head and lifting the chin.
- Assess breathing and pulse for no more than 10 seconds.

3. **Calling for help** :

    - If cardiorespiratory arrest is confirmed, call emergency services immediately (appropriate emergency number).

4. **Cardiopulmonary resuscitation (CPR)** :

    - **Chest compressions**: Place your hands in the center of the chest, between the two nipples, and perform compressions to a depth of 5 to 6 cm, at a frequency of 100 to 120 compressions per minute.
    - **Ventilations**: After 30 compressions, administer 2 insufflations by pinching the nose and blowing air into the patient's mouth, observing the chest rise.
    - Continue the cycle of 30 compressions for 2 breaths until help arrives or signs of life return.

5. **Using the automatic external defibrillator (AED)** :

    - If available, switch on the AED and follow the voice instructions.
    - Place the electrodes on the patient's chest as shown.
    - Make sure no one touches the patient during rhythm analysis and shock delivery, if recommended.
    - Resume CPR immediately after the shock, or if no shock is advised.

Importance of early CPR

Every minute without CPR reduces the chances of survival by 7-10%. Rapid intervention by a bystander can double or even triple the chances of survival. CPR maintains minimal blood flow to preserve vital organs while waiting for advanced care.

Advanced life support

When medical help arrives, additional interventions are carried out:

- **Airway management**: Tracheal intubation to ensure effective ventilation.
- **Administration of medication**: Epinephrine, amiodarone or others according to protocols and identified heart rhythm.
- **Monitoring and diagnosis**: cardiac monitoring, blood gases, identification and treatment of reversible causes (the "4 H's and 4 T's").

The "4 H's and 4 T's": Reversible causes of cardiorespiratory arrest

1. **Hypoxia**
2. **Hypovolemia**
3. **Hypo/hyperkalemia and metabolic disorders**
4. **Hypothermia**
5. **Cardiac tamponade**
6. **Toxics**
7. **Pulmonary thrombosis (pulmonary embolism)**

8. Coronary thrombosis (myocardial infarction)

Rapid identification of these causes enables specific treatments to be put in place to restore cardiac activity.

Prognosis and factors influencing survival

The prognosis depends on several factors:

- **Time to start CPR**: The faster the intervention, the better the chances of survival without neurological sequelae.
- **Cause of stoppage**: Some causes have a better prognosis if they are quickly corrected.
- **Quality of CPR**: Effective, continuous chest compressions are essential.
- **Duration of stoppage**: Prolonged stoppage without effective circulation reduces the chances of neurological recovery.

Preventing cardiorespiratory arrest

Prevention involves managing cardiovascular risk factors and recognizing early warning signs:

- **Control of hypertension**, diabetes and dyslipidemia.
- **Stop smoking** and limit alcohol consumption.
- **A balanced diet** and regular physical activity.
- **Recognizing heart attack symptoms**: Chest pain, shortness of breath, cold sweat.
- **Public education**: Training in first aid and AED use.

Psychological and social impact

Cardiorespiratory arrest has a considerable impact on the surviving patient and those around him:

- **Rehabilitation**: Survivors may require cardiac and neurological rehabilitation.
- **Psychological support**: to deal with anxiety, depression or post-traumatic stress.
- **Family implications**: Loved ones may also need support to deal with the emotional consequences.

The role of the first witnesses

Training the general public in first aid is crucial. Witnesses of cardiorespiratory arrest are the first actors in the chain of survival:

- **CPR training**: Short, accessible courses teach life-saving gestures.
- **Access to AEDs**: The proliferation of AEDs in public places increases the chances of early defibrillation.

Technological advances and research

Medical progress continues to improve the management of cardiorespiratory arrest:

- **Circulatory assistance devices**: ECMO (extracorporeal membrane oxygenation) can be used in some cases to maintain circulation.
- **Artificial intelligence algorithms**: to improve recognition of cardiac arrest by emergency services.
- **Pharmacological research**: Development of new drugs to optimize resuscitation.

- Falls and injuries

Falls and the resulting injuries are a major public health problem affecting people of all ages, although children and the elderly are particularly vulnerable. These incidents can result in injuries ranging from minor to serious, or even fatal. Understanding the causes of falls, identifying risk factors and implementing preventive measures are essential to reduce their incidence and mitigate their consequences on individual and collective health.

Understanding falls

A fall is defined as an event in which a person involuntarily lands on the ground or at a lower level than where they were initially standing. Trauma resulting from falls can be physical, psychological and social. Physical injuries include contusions, fractures, head trauma and soft tissue damage. Psychological consequences can include a fear of falling again, leading to reduced mobility and independence. Socially, falls can lead to isolation and reduced quality of life.

Causes and risk factors for falls

Several factors, often interconnected, increase the risk of falling:

1. **Individual factors** :
   - **Advanced age**: Aging is accompanied by a decline in muscle strength, balance and coordination.
   - **Health problems**: Chronic illnesses such as arthritis, Parkinson's disease, vision problems or orthostatic hypotension increase the risk of falling.
   - **Medications**: Some treatments, especially sedatives, antihypertensives or diuretics, can cause dizziness or reduced alertness.
   - **Cognitive impairment**: Cognitive impairment or dementia can affect judgment and the ability to assess environmental risks.

2. **Environmental factors** :

    - **Household obstacles**: Slippery carpets, electrical cables on the floor, inadequate lighting or stairs without handrails all increase the risk in the home.
    - **Outdoor conditions**: Uneven sidewalks, wet ground, snow or black ice are all risk factors in public spaces.
    - **Unsuitable footwear**: Wearing uncomfortable, slippery or high-heeled shoes increases the risk of falling.

3. **Risky behavior** :

    - **Dangerous activities**: Climbing on unstable chairs to reach high objects.
    - **Alcohol or drug use**: Impaired balance and coordination due to these substances increase the risk of falling.

Consequences of falls and trauma

Falls can result in a variety of injuries, the severity of which depends on factors such as the height of the fall, the impact surface, body position and the person's state of health:

- **Bone fractures**: especially of hips, wrists, arms and ankles.
- **Head injuries**: From concussion to intracranial hemorrhage.
- **Soft tissue injuries**: Contusions, sprains, muscle or ligament tears.
- **Death**: Falls are a major cause of accidental death, especially among the elderly.

Psychological consequences include :

- **Fear of falling**: Can lead to activity limitation, aggravating muscle weakness and increasing the risk of further falls.
- **Loss of self-confidence**: Impact on quality of life and emotional well-being.

Falls and trauma prevention

Prevention requires a multidimensional approach, integrating individual, environmental and societal interventions.

1. **Individual risk assessment and management :**

    - **Regular medical check-ups**: Detection and treatment of health problems contributing to falls.
    - **Medication review**: Assessment to minimize fall-related side effects.
    - **Improving physical condition**:
        - **Balance and muscle-strengthening exercises**: Programs such as tai chi, gentle gymnastics or physiotherapy.
        - **Regular physical activity**: Walking, swimming or cycling to maintain mobility and muscle strength.

2. **Adapting to the environment :**

    - **Home security :**
        - **Adequate lighting**: Adequate lighting in all rooms and passageways.
        - **Removing obstacles**: removing slippery carpets, storing objects on the floor, securing cables.

- **Assistive equipment**: Grab bars in the bathroom, handrails on stairs, non-slip shower seats.
  - **Safety in public spaces** :
    - **Maintenance of sidewalks and footpaths**: repair of uneven surfaces, snow removal, marking of hazardous areas.

3. **Education and awareness** :
   - **Community programs**: Workshops on falls prevention, information on risks and preventive measures.
   - **Training healthcare professionals**: To identify people at risk and propose appropriate interventions.
   - **Awareness campaigns**: promoting home safety and preventive behavior.

4. **Use of technical aids** :
   - **Walking aids**: walking sticks, walkers for people with balance or mobility problems.
   - **Suitable footwear**: Wear comfortable, well-fitting shoes with non-slip soles.

Falls and trauma management

In the event of a fall, rapid and appropriate intervention is essential to limit complications:

1. **Initial assessment** :
   - **Ensure safety**: Avoid moving the person if serious injury is suspected.
   - **Check state of consciousness**: Assess breathing, pulse, reaction to stimuli.

- **Call for help**: In case of serious injury, loss of consciousness or severe pain.

2. **First aid** :

    - **Control bleeding**: Apply pressure to open wounds.
    - **Immobilization**: Do not mobilize a limb suspected of being fractured; use splints if trained to do so.
    - **Ice application**: on bruised areas to reduce inflammation and pain.

3. **Medical follow-up** :

    - **Medical consultation**: assess the extent of injuries, carry out additional tests (X-rays, scans).
    - **Rehabilitation**: Physiotherapy to restore mobility, strengthen muscles and prevent future falls.
    - **Psychological support**: Helping people overcome their fear of falling back.

Societal and economic impact of falls

Falls have a significant impact on the healthcare system and society:

- **High medical costs**: hospitalization, surgery, rehabilitation.
- **Loss of autonomy**: Increased need for assistance at home or admission to a specialized facility.
- **Burden on caregivers**: Stress and exhaustion for relatives caring for people who have suffered a fall.

First aid and emergency procedures

- Cardiopulmonary resuscitation (CPR)

Cardiopulmonary resuscitation (CPR) is an emergency life-saving technique designed to maintain blood circulation and organ oxygenation in the event of cardiac arrest. It consists of a series of maneuvers designed to temporarily replace the action of the heart and lungs until vital functions can be restored, either spontaneously or through advanced medical intervention. CPR is an essential skill that everyone should master, as rapid intervention can double or even triple a cardiac arrest victim's chances of survival.

Importance of CPR

Every year, thousands of people suffer sudden cardiac arrest, whether at home, at work or in public places. Cardiac arrest is a critical situation in which the heart stops pumping blood, depriving the brain and vital organs of oxygen. Without immediate intervention, irreversible brain damage can occur within minutes, rapidly leading to death. CPR maintains minimal blood flow to the brain and heart, prolonging the window of survival until medical help arrives.

Signs of cardiac arrest

To react effectively, it is crucial to recognize the signs of cardiac arrest quickly:

- **Loss of consciousness**: The victim does not react when spoken to or stimulated.
- **Absence of breathing**: The chest does not rise, no breath is felt.
- **Absence of pulse**: No perceptible heartbeat in the major arteries (carotid or femoral).

CPR steps

CPR follows a precise sequence of actions, often summarized by the A-B-C diagram (Airway, Breathing, Circulation):

1. **Scene safety**
   First and foremost, make sure the environment is safe for you and the victim. Eliminate potential dangers such as traffic, fire or electrical hazards.

2. **Assessing consciousness**
   Approach the victim, gently shake his shoulders and ask loudly: "Can you hear me?". If there is no response, assume the victim is unconscious.

3. **Call for help**
   Shout to attract the attention of people nearby. Specifically ask someone to call the emergency services and, if possible, to bring an automatic external defibrillator (AED).

4. **Opening the airway**
   Lay the victim on his back on a flat, hard surface. Tilt the head back, lifting the chin with two fingers ("chin-front" maneuver) to open the airway.

5. **Checking breathing**
   Bring your cheek close to the victim's mouth, watch for chest rise, listen and feel for any breaths for at least 5 seconds, but no more than 10 seconds. If the victim is not breathing or is breathing abnormally (gasping), start CPR immediately.

6. **Chest compressions**
   - **Hand positioning**: Place the palm of one hand on the center of the chest, on the breastbone, between the two nipples. Place the other hand on top, interlacing the fingers.

- **Technique**: Keep your arms straight, shoulders aligned above your hands, and use your body weight to perform the compressions.
- **Depth and rhythm**: Press down hard to depress the sternum by about 5 to 6 centimetres with each compression. Perform compressions at a rate of 100 to 120 per minute.
- **Release**: Allow the chest to return to its initial position between each compression, without removing your hands.

7. **Ventilation**

    - **After 30 compressions**, perform 2 insufflations:
        - **Pinch the victim's nose** to prevent air from escaping.
        - **Take a normal breath** and seal your lips around her mouth.
        - **Inhale slowly** for about 1 second, checking that the chest rises.
        - **Take another breath** and repeat a second insufflation.
    - Note: If you're not trained in insufflations, or if you're uncomfortable performing them, it's acceptable to perform chest compressions only ("hands-only" CPR).

8. **Continuing CPR**

    Continue the cycle of 30 compressions for 2 breaths without interruption until :

    - The arrival of professional help.
    - The appearance of signs of normal breathing.
    - Rescuer exhaustion.

9. **Using the automatic external defibrillator (AED)**

    ○ **Set-up**: As soon as an AED is available, switch it on and follow the voice instructions.
    ○ **Electrode placement**: Apply the electrodes to the victim's bare chest, one under the right collarbone, the other under the left breast, on the flank.
    ○ **Rhythm analysis**: The AED will analyze the heart rhythm and determine whether a shock is required.
    ○ **Shock administration**: If the AED recommends a shock, make sure no-one is touching the victim and press the shock button.
    ○ **Resuming CPR**: After the shock, resume chest compressions immediately.

Special aspects for children and infants

CPR techniques for children (1 year to puberty) and infants (less than 1 year) have a few differences:

- **Chest compressions** :

    ○ **Children**: Use one or two hands depending on the child's size, pressing down on the center of the chest to depress the sternum by about a third of the thoracic depth.
    ○ **Infants**: Use two fingers (index and middle) in the center of the chest, below the nipple line, and compress one-third of the way down the chest.

- **Ventilation** :

    ○ Perform 5 initial insufflations before starting compressions.

- Cover the infant's mouth and nose with your mouth for insufflations.

Importance of CPR training

Although instructions can be followed in an emergency situation, practical CPR training is highly recommended. These courses, often offered by first-aid associations, enable you to acquire the correct gestures, practice on mannequins and gain the confidence to act effectively in a real emergency.

Barriers to intervention and how to overcome them

- **Fear of doing the wrong thing**: It's better to try something than to do nothing. Even imperfect CPR increases the chances of survival.
- **Legal risk**: Laws generally protect citizens who act in good faith to help someone in danger.
- **Apprehension about insufflations**: If you're reluctant, give preference to continuous chest compressions.

The chain of survival

Successful management of cardiac arrest is based on a series of coordinated actions known as the "chain of survival":

1. **Early recognition and call for help**: Identify cardiac arrest and quickly alert emergency services.
2. **Immediate start of CPR**: Provide quality chest compressions to maintain blood flow.
3. **Rapid defibrillation**: Use an AED as soon as possible to restore a normal heart rhythm.
4. **Advanced care**: Administration of specialized medical care by healthcare professionals.
5. **Post-cardiac arrest resuscitation**: in-hospital management to treat underlying causes and prevent complications.

Preventing cardiac arrest

- **Adopt a healthy lifestyle**: regular physical activity, balanced diet, stop smoking.
- **Controlling risk factors**: monitoring blood pressure, cholesterol and diabetes.
- **Public education**: Raising awareness of the warning signs of myocardial infarction and stroke.
- **Access to defibrillators**: Installation of AEDs in public places and training in their use.

- Lateral safety position (PLS)

The lateral position of safety (PLS) is an essential first-aid technique which consists of placing an unconscious but spontaneously breathing person on his or her side, in order to keep the airway clear and prevent the risk of asphyxia. This simple maneuver can save lives by preventing the tongue or fluids such as blood, saliva or vomit from obstructing the airway. Understanding when and how to apply PLS is essential for anyone involved in emergency rescue.

The importance of PLS in first aid

When a person loses consciousness, muscle tone drops considerably. The tongue, a supple muscle, can then fall back towards the back of the throat and obstruct the airway, preventing air from flowing freely to the lungs. In addition, lying on the back increases the risk of inhalation of body fluids, which can lead to asphyxia or aspiration pneumonia. PLS mitigates these risks by positioning the victim in such a way as to keep the airways open and facilitate the outflow of fluids.

When to use the lateral position

PLS must be applied in the following situations:

- The victim is unconscious but breathing normally.

- There is no suspicion of trauma to the spine, particularly the cervical spine.
- Wait for emergency medical services to arrive, after alerting the emergency services.

It's crucial to always assess the person's state of consciousness and breathing before intervening. If the victim is not breathing or has abnormal breathing (gasping), cardiopulmonary resuscitation (CPR) should be started immediately, rather than placing the victim in the SCP position.

Steps for the lateral safety position

PLS positioning must be carried out with care to avoid aggravating possible injuries. Here are the detailed steps for correctly positioning a person in PLS:

1. **Make the scene safe**
   Before approaching the victim, check that the environment is safe for you and the victim. Eliminate potential hazards such as traffic, fire or dangerous objects.

2. **Assess state of consciousness**
   Approach the victim, speak loudly and clearly: "Can you hear me? Open your eyes!" If she doesn't respond, gently shake her shoulders to stimulate a reaction. Failure to respond indicates loss of consciousness.

3. **Check breathing**
   Gently open the airway by tilting the head back slightly and lifting the chin. Bring your ear close to his mouth and look towards his chest for at least 10 seconds to :
   - **See** if the chest rises.
   - **Hearing** a breath.
   - **Feel** the air on your cheek.

4. If breathing is normal, you can perform PLS. If not, immediately call for help and start CPR.

5. **Call for help**
   Ask someone to call the emergency services (15 for the SAMU in France, 112 for the European emergency number), or do it yourself if you're alone. Give precise information about the victim's location and condition.

6. **Preparing the victim for PLS**

    - **Remove glasses** if worn.
    - **Check the pockets** to remove any objects that may cause discomfort during positioning.

7. **Position the nearest arm**

    - Place the victim's arm on your side at right angles to their body, elbow bent, palm up.

8. **Preparing the other arm**

    - Take the victim's opposite arm and place it on his chest, resting the back of his hand against his opposite cheek (closest to you).

9. **Bend opposite leg**

    - Grab the opposite leg (furthest from you) just above the knee and bend it, foot flat on the floor, keeping the foot in contact with the ground.

10. **Roll the victim onto his side**

    - Holding the victim's hand against his cheek, gently pull on the bent leg to rotate the body towards you, until it's on its side.

11. **Adjust position**

    - Adjust the upper leg so that the hip and knee are at right angles. This ensures a stable position.

- Tilt the head back slightly to keep the airway open.
- Open the victim's mouth to allow fluids to drain away.
- Check that the hand under the cheek keeps the head in a neutral position.

12. Continuous monitoring

- Stay with the victim until help arrives.
- Regularly check your breathing by observing the movement of your chest.
- If the victim is to remain in the PLS position for a prolonged period, turn him onto his other side every 30 minutes to avoid pressure points.

Special precautions

- **Suspected cervical or spinal trauma**: If you suspect a spinal injury (for example, after a road accident or a fall from a height), it's best not to move the victim to avoid aggravating a spinal injury. However, if the person is vomiting or having difficulty breathing, it may be necessary to place him/her in the supine position with extreme caution.

- **Pregnant women**: If the victim is more than 6 months pregnant, we recommend placing her on her left side to avoid compression of the inferior vena cava by the uterus, which could compromise venous return to the heart.

The importance of first aid training

Although PLS is a relatively simple technique, practical first aid training is highly recommended to acquire the necessary skills and react effectively in an emergency situation. Training courses, provided by accredited organizations, teach how to :

- Correctly assess a victim's condition.
- Apply the appropriate gestures according to the situation.
- Use an automatic external defibrillator (AED).
- Manage stress and communicate effectively with emergency services.

- Using the automated external defibrillator (AED)

The Automated External Defibrillator (AED) is a portable medical device designed to analyze the heart rhythm of a person in sudden cardiac arrest and, if necessary, deliver an electric shock to restore normal heart rhythm. The rapid and appropriate use of an AED, combined with high-quality cardiopulmonary resuscitation (CPR), significantly increases the victim's chances of survival. Understanding how an AED works and knowing how to use it is essential for everyone, because cardiac arrest can happen anywhere, at any time.

Understanding sudden cardiac arrest

Sudden cardiac arrest is a critical medical condition in which the heart abruptly stops pumping blood, resulting in loss of consciousness and the absence of normal breathing. The most common causes are heart rhythm abnormalities, notably ventricular fibrillation, where the heart's electrical impulses become chaotic. Without immediate intervention, cardiac arrest rapidly leads to irreversible brain damage and death.

Importance of the automated external defibrillator

The AED plays a crucial role in the chain of survival. It enables non-medical personnel to intervene rapidly in the event of cardiac arrest. Every minute that passes without defibrillation reduces the chances of survival by 7-10%. Early intervention with an AED can double or even triple the chances of survival.

DAE operation

The AED is designed to be easy to use. It generally includes :

- **An ignition button**: to start the appliance.
- **Adhesive electrodes**: To be placed on the victim's bare chest.
- **Voice and visual instructions**: to guide the user through the process.

The AED automatically analyzes the victim's heart rhythm and determines whether a shock is required. It delivers a shock only when indicated, avoiding any risk of misuse.

Steps for using an AED

1. **Ensure scene safety**
   Before intervening, check that the environment is safe for you and the victim. Eliminate potential hazards such as water sources, electrical hazards or road traffic.

2. **Check the victim's condition**
   - **Awareness assessment**: Gently shake the person's shoulders and ask aloud, "Can you hear me?"
   - **Check breathing**: If the victim doesn't respond, open the airway by tilting the head back and lifting the chin. Look, listen and feel for normal breathing for at least 5 seconds, but no more than 10.

3. **Call for help**
   - **Ask someone to call the emergency services** (15 for the SAMU in France, 112 for the European emergency number) and bring back an AED if available.
   - If you are alone, call for help yourself before starting resuscitation.

4. **Starting cardiopulmonary resuscitation (CPR)**
    - **Chest compressions**: Place your hands in the center of the victim's chest and begin compressions at a rate of 100 to 120 per minute.
    - **Alternate with insufflations**: If you are trained, after 30 compressions, administer 2 insufflations.

5. **Switch on the AED as soon as it is available**
    - **Switching on**: Press the unit's ignition button.
    - **Follow instructions**: The AED will guide you vocally and/or visually.

6. **Preparing the victim for defibrillation**
    - **Exposing the chest**: Open or remove clothing to gain access to bare skin.
    - **Dry the skin if necessary**: If the chest is wet, dry it quickly to ensure good electrode adhesion.
    - **Shave if possible**: If hair growth is excessive and a razor is provided, quickly shave the area where the electrodes will be placed.

7. **Place electrodes**
    - **Electrode 1**: Place it under the victim's right clavicle, just below the collarbone.
    - **Electrode 2**: Place it on the left side of the chest, under the left armpit, a few centimetres below the nipple.

8. **Analyze heart rate**
    - **Make sure no one touches the victim** during the analysis.

- The **AED will automatically analyze** the heart rhythm and determine whether a shock is required.

9. **Delivering shock**

    - **If the AED recommends a shock** :
        - **Check again that no one is touching the victim**.
        - **Press the shock button** if the AED is not fully automatic.
        - **Some AEDs deliver the shock** automatically after a countdown.

10. **Resume CPR**

    - **Immediately after shock**, resume chest compressions.
    - **Follow the AED's instructions**, which may tell you to continue CPR for two minutes before a new scan.

11. **Continue until help arrives**

    - **Continue CPR and defibrillation cycles** as indicated by the AED.
    - **Stop manoeuvring only if** :
        - The victim resumes normal breathing and shows signs of life.
        - Professional rescue services take over.
        - You're exhausted and unable to continue.

Precautions when using the AED

- **Wet environment**: Avoid using the AED if the victim is immersed in water. Move to a dry area if possible.

- **Metal surface**: If the victim is on a metal surface, make sure the electrodes are not in contact with the metal to avoid electrical hazards.
- **Presence of pacemaker**: If the victim has a visible pacemaker (small bump under the skin), place the electrodes at least a few centimetres away from it.

Myths and facts about AEDs

- "**I can hurt the victim**": The AED is designed to be safe. It will only administer a shock if necessary.
- "**I could be electrocuted**": If you follow the precautions (don't touch the victim during the shock), the risk is minimal.
- "**I'm not trained, I can't use it**": AEDs are designed for the general public. Voice instructions guide you step by step.

Importance of training

Although AEDs are easy to use, training in first aid and AED use is highly recommended. This will enable you to:

- **Act with confidence** in emergency situations.
- **Practice CPR techniques** to ensure effective compressions.
- **Learn to recognize the signs** of cardiac arrest and other medical emergencies.

Deployment of AEDs in public places

Many countries have set up programs to install AEDs in public places, such as :

- Airports
- Shopping centers
- The stations

- The stadiums
- The companies

Publicly accessible AEDs are essential for rapid intervention.

Role of emergency services

When you call the emergency services :

- **Clearly indicate your location.**
- **Inform them that you are with a victim in cardiac arrest** and that you are using an AED.
- **Follow any instructions** they may give you over the phone.

After using the AED

- **Leave electrodes in place**: professional rescuers may need to continue defibrillation.
- **Inform the rescue team** of everything you've done: number of shocks delivered, time elapsed, observations.

Psychological impact

Intervening in an emergency situation can be stressful. After the incident :

- **Take care of yourself**: Talk about your experience with loved ones or professionals if necessary.
- **Know that your intervention has made a difference**: whatever the outcome, your action is precious.

Alert and Reporting Procedures

- Rapid communication with the medical team

Fast, efficient communication with the medical team is a crucial element in ensuring quality patient care. In a healthcare environment where every second counts, the accurate and timely transmission of information can mean the difference between life and death. This communication is not limited to the exchange of clinical information, but also encompasses the coordination of efforts, shared decision-making and the creation of a collaborative environment conducive to excellence in care.

The importance of rapid communication

Speed of communication is essential for several reasons:

1. **Reactivity to emergencies**: In critical situations such as cardiac arrest, respiratory distress or major haemorrhage, immediate communication enables us to mobilize the necessary resources quickly and initiate the appropriate interventions.

2. **Preventing medical errors**: Communication errors are a major cause of adverse events. Fast, clear transmission of information reduces the risk of misunderstandings, duplications or omissions in care.

3. **Multidisciplinary coordination**: Patient care often involves several healthcare professionals. Fluid communication between doctors, nurses, pharmacists and others ensures consistent, effective care.

4. **Adapting to clinical changes**: A patient's condition can evolve rapidly. Promptly informing the medical team of changes enables the care plan to be adjusted accordingly.

Principles of effective communication

To ensure that communication is not only rapid but also effective, certain fundamental principles must be respected:

1. **Clarity**: Messages should be precise, concise and unambiguous. The use of common language and the avoidance of unnecessary jargon facilitate understanding.

2. **Relevance**: Convey essential information relevant to the clinical situation. Avoid superfluous details that may dilute the main message.

3. **Structure**: Organize information logically. Tools such as the SBAR (Situation, Background, Assessment, Recommendation) protocol can help structure communication.

4. **Assertiveness**: Clearly express observations, concerns and recommendations, while respecting the opinions of other team members.

5. **Active listening**: Pay attention to the listener's answers and concerns, encouraging dialogue and questions to clarify unclear points.

Methods and tools for rapid communication

Several methods and tools can facilitate rapid communication with the medical team:

1. **Information and communication technologies (ICT)** :

    - **Secure instant messaging systems**: Enable messages to be sent quickly to team members, while respecting the confidentiality of medical data.

- **Mobile applications**: Provide real-time access to electronic medical records, laboratory results and medical images.
- **Alerts and notifications**: integrated alarm systems instantly alert caregivers to critical changes in the patient's condition.

2. **Short, regular team meetings** :

    - **Briefings**: Short exchanges at the start of each shift to share key information and priorities for the day.
    - **Debriefings**: Discussions after a critical event to analyze actions, identify areas for improvement and strengthen collaboration.

3. **Standardized communication protocols** :

    - **SBAR**: Facilitates the structured transmission of information during handovers or inter-professional consultations.
    - **Checklists**: Ensure that all important information is communicated and essential procedures followed.

4. **Visual dashboards** :

    - **Information panels**: Display key patient data, tasks and responsibilities.
    - **Performance indicators**: Track progress and highlight areas requiring particular attention.

The challenges of rapid communication

Despite the advantages, several challenges can hamper rapid communication:

1. **Information overload**: The high volume of data can overwhelm caregivers, making it difficult to identify crucial information.

2. **Technological barriers**: computer system malfunctions or lack of compatibility between platforms can slow down communication.

3. **Resistance to change**: Some professionals may be reluctant to adopt new communication methods or technologies.

4. **Time constraints**: Emergencies and workloads can limit the time available for effective communication.

Strategies for overcoming challenges

1. **Training and education** :

    - **Communication workshops**: Developing interpersonal communication skills and the use of technological tools.
    - **Protocol awareness**: Train staff in standardized methods such as SBAR.

2. **Improving technological systems** :

    - **Investment in reliable infrastructure**: Ensuring regular system maintenance and software updates.
    - **Systems integration**: Promote interoperability between different platforms for seamless communication.

3. **Promoting a collaborative culture** :

    - **Participative leadership**: encourage managers to model open communication and value the contributions of every team member.

- **Recognition of efforts**: Celebrate successes and improvements resulting from effective communication.

4. **Time management** :

    - **Prioritize tasks**: Identify essential activities that require immediate communication.
    - **Resource allocation**: Delegate certain responsibilities to allow caregivers to focus on critical communications.

The impact of rapid communication on patient care

Fast, effective communication has a direct positive impact on the quality of care:

1. **Improved patient safety**: Reduced medication errors, treatment delays and avoidable complications.

2. **Optimized clinical outcomes**: earlier intervention in the face of clinical deterioration, leading to better prognosis.

3. **Patient and family satisfaction**: A coordinated, responsive team strengthens patient confidence in the care system.

4. **Operational efficiency**: Fluid communication improves resource management, reduces redundancies and speeds up decision-making processes.

The role of technology in facilitating communication

Technological advances offer new opportunities to improve communication:

1. **Electronic medical records (EMR)**: centralize patient information, accessible in real time by all team members.

2. **Telecommunications and telemedicine**: enable remote consultations, rapid expert advice and patient follow-up outside healthcare establishments.

3. **Artificial intelligence and predictive alerts**: Analyze data to anticipate potential complications and warn the medical team in advance.

- Incident documentation

Incident documentation is an essential element in the effective management of organizations, particularly in sectors where safety, quality and compliance are paramount. It involves the detailed recording of all undesirable events, accidents, near misses or malfunctions that occur within an organization. The aim of this practice is to analyze these incidents in order to understand their root causes, learn from them and put in place corrective measures to avoid their recurrence. Rigorous incident documentation not only helps to improve safety and performance, but also reinforces a culture of transparency and accountability within the organization.

Importance of incident documentation

1. **Continuous improvement**: Documentation helps identify weaknesses and vulnerabilities in operational processes. By analyzing incidents, organizations can implement targeted improvements to strengthen their systems and procedures.

2. **Preventing future incidents**: By understanding the underlying causes of incidents, preventive strategies can be developed. This not only reduces safety risks, but also the costs associated with downtime and repairs.

3. **Regulatory compliance**: Many industries are subject to strict regulations that require detailed incident records to be kept. Proper documentation is essential to demonstrate compliance with legal and industry standards.

4. **Accountability and transparency**: Documentation fosters a culture where employees are encouraged to report incidents without fear of negative repercussions. This fosters open communication and collective awareness of safety and quality issues.

5. **Training and awareness**: Incident reports can be used as educational tools to train staff in best practices and lessons learned, reinforcing team skills and vigilance.

Key elements of effective documentation

1. **Detailed information gathering**

    - **Date, time and place**: Indicate precisely when and where the incident occurred.
    - **Incident description**: Provide a clear, factual account of what happened, without subjective interpretation.
    - **People involved**: Name the individuals affected or witnesses, while respecting confidentiality rules.
    - **Surrounding conditions**: Note specific circumstances, such as weather conditions, equipment status or operational context.
    - **Immediate consequences**: Describe direct impacts, such as injuries, property damage or service interruptions.

2. **Analysis of causes**

    - **Identification of immediate causes**: Determine the factors that led directly to the incident.
    - **Root cause review**: Explore underlying reasons, such as procedural shortcomings, inadequate training or organizational problems.

- **Use of analysis methods**: Apply tools such as the Ishikawa diagram (cause and effect) or the "5 whys" method to deepen the analysis.

3. **Corrective and preventive actions**

    - **Action planning**: Establish specific actions to remedy identified causes.
    - **Assigned responsibilities**: Designate individuals or teams to implement measures.
    - **Deadlines**: Set realistic deadlines for completing actions.
    - **Monitoring and evaluation**: Set up indicators to measure the effectiveness of measures and adjust if necessary.

4. **Structured, accessible documentation**

    - **Use of standardized forms**: Facilitate consistency and comparability of reports.
    - **Secure storage**: Ensure that documents are stored in a reliable, protected system.
    - **Controlled access**: Allow authorized persons to access information while protecting confidentiality.

5. **Communication and feedback**

    - **Sharing lessons learned**: Disseminate relevant information to the relevant teams to prevent future incidents.
    - **Employee feedback**: Encourage suggestions and comments to improve documentation and incident management processes.

Challenges and obstacles to incident documentation

1. **Reluctance to report incidents**

- **Blame culture**: If employees fear sanctions, they may be reluctant to report incidents.
- **Lack of awareness**: A lack of understanding of the importance of documentation can reduce participation.

2. **Administrative burden**

    - **Process complexity**: Overly cumbersome or complicated procedures can discourage staff.
    - **Limited resources** : Lack of time or dedicated staff can hamper proper documentation.

3. **Data management**

    - **Information overload**: A massive influx of data can make analysis difficult.
    - **Quality of information** : Incomplete or inaccurate reports compromise the usefulness of documentation.

Strategies for improving incident documentation

1. **Promoting a positive culture**

    - **Encourage reporting**: Value employees who report incidents, emphasizing the importance for collective safety.
    - **Training and awareness**: Organize sessions to explain procedures and the impact of documentation on improving practices.

2. **Process simplification**

    - **User-friendly forms**: Design simple, intuitive reporting tools.
    - **Technology integration**: Use digital platforms to facilitate data capture and processing.

3. **Management commitment**

    - **Exemplary leadership**: Managers must set an example by actively supporting documentation initiatives.
    - **Adequate resources** : Allocate the necessary resources to ensure effective incident management.

4. **Proactive data analysis**

    - **Advanced analytical tools**: Set up systems to process and interpret data efficiently.
    - **Performance indicators**: Define metrics to monitor trends and evaluate improvements.

Impact of incident documentation on the organization

1. **Enhanced safety**

    - **Reducing accidents**: Preventive measures reduce the number and severity of incidents.
    - **Improved well-being**: A safer environment increases employee satisfaction and productivity.

2. **Process optimization**

    - **Operational efficiency**: Identifying inefficiencies leads to improvements in procedures and systems.
    - **Innovation**: Lessons learned from incidents can stimulate creativity and the adoption of new approaches.

3. **Image and reputation**

    ○ **Stakeholder confidence**: Transparent incident management enhances credibility with customers, partners and regulators.
    ○ **Competitive advantage**: Organizations that demonstrate a strong commitment to safety and quality can stand out in the marketplace.

- Participation in post-incident debriefings

Participation in post-incident debriefings is an indispensable practice in many professional fields, including healthcare, public safety, the military and industry. It involves bringing team members together after a critical or unusual event to collectively analyze what happened, learn from it and improve future practices. This approach not only contributes to the continuous improvement of processes, but also provides psychological support for those involved and strengthens team cohesion.

Importance of post-incident debriefings

Debriefings provide a valuable opportunity to reflect on incidents, whether successes or failures. They enable :

- **Analyze actions taken**: Understand what has worked well and identify areas for improvement.
- **Sharing experiences**: Each member can contribute his or her own unique point of view, enriching collective understanding.
- **Strengthen communication**: Open, honest dialogue is essential for effective collaboration.
- **Supporting responders' well-being**: Provide a space to express emotions, reduce post-traumatic stress and prevent burnout.

Benefits of active participation

1. **Learning and continuous improvement**
   Participation in debriefings helps identify gaps in procedures, training or resources. By discussing the challenges encountered and possible solutions, teams can adapt their practices to be better prepared for the future.

2. **Strengthening team cohesion**
   Sharing difficult or intense experiences creates bonds between team members. Mutual recognition of each other's efforts and contributions fosters trust and respect, key elements of harmonious collaboration.

3. **Personal and professional development**
   Debriefings provide an opportunity for personal reflection on one's own performance. Participants can receive constructive feedback, identify their strengths and areas for development, thus contributing to their professional growth.

4. **Managing emotions and stress**
   Expressing your feelings in a safe environment helps you process the emotions associated with the incident. This reduces the risk of psychological disorders such as anxiety, depression or post-traumatic stress.

Principles of effective debriefing

For participation in debriefings to be beneficial, certain conditions must be met:

1. **Creating a safe environment**
   It is essential that participants feel comfortable expressing themselves without fear of judgment or reprisal. Confidentiality and mutual respect must be guaranteed.

2. **Open and honest communication**
Encourage the free expression of opinions, concerns and suggestions. Exchanges should focus on facts and processes, rather than individuals.

3. **Structured approach**
Using a framework or methodology to guide debriefing helps to cover all relevant aspects. Models such as "SAFER" (Support, Analysis, Facts, Emotions, Summary) or "DESC" (Describe, Express, Specify, Consequences) can be useful.

4. **Focus on learning**
The main objective is to learn from experience in order to improve future practices. It's important to avoid the search for culprits and focus on solutions.

Role of participants

- **Facilitator**
A trained facilitator or moderator can lead the debriefing, ensuring that the discussion remains productive and that all participants have the opportunity to express themselves.

- **Team members**
Each participant brings a unique perspective. It's important that they are engaged, actively listen and contribute constructively.

Potential challenges and solutions

1. **Emotional barriers**
Critical incidents can arouse strong emotions. It's important to recognize these feelings and provide appropriate support, possibly with the help of mental health professionals.

2. **Blame culture**
   If participants fear blame, they will be less inclined to share openly. Promoting a just culture, where the emphasis is on learning rather than punishment, is essential.

3. **Lack of time**
   Operational constraints can make it difficult to organize debriefings. However, it is important to prioritize these moments for the long-term benefits they bring.

4. **Diversity of participants**
   Differences in culture, language or hierarchical level can affect group dynamics. Adapting the approach to include all members and promote equality of speech is crucial.

Strategies for optimizing participation

- **Training and awareness**
  Training teams in debriefing techniques and the importance of these sessions can improve commitment and efficiency.

- **Process integration**
  Making debriefings a standard part of procedures after every incident reinforces their importance and regularity.

- **Use of technology**
  In some cases, digital tools can facilitate participation, especially for geographically dispersed teams.

- **Continuous feedback**
  Soliciting feedback from participants on the debriefing process enables us to constantly improve the process.

Chapter 6

Palliative and End-of-Life Care

Principles of Palliative Care

- Pain and symptom relief

Pain and its associated symptoms are a daily reality for many people suffering from acute or chronic illnesses. Relieving these discomforts is essential to improving patients' quality of life, promoting their well-being and facilitating their participation in daily activities. A holistic and personalized approach is often required to effectively manage pain and symptoms, taking into account the physical, emotional and social dimensions of each individual.

Understanding pain and symptoms

Pain is an unpleasant sensory and emotional experience associated with actual or potential tissue damage. It can be acute, occurring suddenly in response to an injury, or chronic, persisting for months or even years. Symptoms, meanwhile, encompass a variety of manifestations such as fatigue, nausea, dyspnea, anxiety and depression, which can accompany a variety of medical conditions.

Importance of pain and symptom relief

Effective pain and symptom control is crucial for several reasons:

1. **Improved quality of life**: Proper management enables patients to lead more active and satisfying lives.

2. **Promoting healing**: By reducing stress and discomfort, the body can better concentrate on healing processes.

3. **Preventing complications**: Uncontrolled pain can lead to problems such as insomnia, depression or reduced immune function.

4. **Respecting patients' rights**: Pain relief is a fundamental aspect of patient-centered care and medical ethics.

Approaches to pain relief

Pain management is based on a combination of pharmacological and non-pharmacological treatments, tailored to the specific needs of each patient.

1. **Pharmacological treatments**

    - **Non-opioid analgesics**: Include paracetamol and non-steroidal anti-inflammatory drugs (NSAIDs) such as ibuprofen. They are effective for mild to moderate pain.

    - **Weak and strong opioids**: Used for moderate to severe pain. Weak opioids include codeine and tramadol, while strong opioids include morphine, oxycodone and fentanyl.

    - **Analgesic adjuvants**: Drugs not originally designed for pain, such as certain antidepressants or anticonvulsants, which may be useful for neuropathic pain.

    - **Local anesthetics and nerve blocks**: Injection of anesthetic drugs to interrupt the transmission of pain signals.

2. **Non-pharmacological treatments**

    - **Physical therapies**: Physiotherapy, massage, application of heat or cold, exercises to strengthen muscles and improve mobility.

- **Cognitive-behavioral techniques**: help patients modify their perception of pain and develop coping strategies.

- **Relaxation and meditation**: Techniques such as deep breathing, mindfulness meditation or yoga to reduce stress and muscle tension.

- **Acupuncture and other complementary therapies**: May offer additional relief for some patients.

Managing associated symptoms

In addition to pain, patients may experience a variety of symptoms that affect their well-being. An integrated approach is needed to manage them effectively.

1. **Fatigue**

    - **Balance between rest and activity**: Plan regular rest periods while maintaining an appropriate level of activity.

    - **Balanced nutrition**: Ensuring an adequate supply of nutrients to sustain energy.

    - **Sleep management**: Establish a healthy sleep routine to improve the quality of night-time rest.

2. **Nausea and vomiting**

    - **Antiemetic drugs**: Prescribed to control nausea induced by treatments such as chemotherapy.

    - **Dietary modifications**: Eat small, frequent meals, avoid fatty or spicy foods.

- **Relaxation techniques**: Can help reduce nausea of psychological origin.

3. **Dyspnea (difficulty breathing)**

    - **Respiratory therapy**: Exercises to improve lung function.
    - **Oxygen therapy**: Administration of oxygen to increase blood oxygen saturation.
    - **Medication**: Bronchodilators or anxiolytics to relieve shortness of breath.

4. **Anxiety and depression**

    - **Psychotherapy**: Individual or group therapy to treat emotional disorders.
    - **Psychotropic medications**: Antidepressants or anxiolytics as required.
    - **Social support**: Participation in support groups, involvement of family and friends.

The role of healthcare professionals

Doctors, nurses, pharmacists and other professionals play a key role in relieving pain and symptoms:

- **Regular assessment**: Use of pain scales and questionnaires to monitor the evolution of symptoms.
- **Care planning**: Development of a personalized treatment plan in collaboration with the patient.
- **Patient education**: providing information on treatment options, side effects and self-management strategies.

- **Follow-up and adjustment**: Regularly reassess the effectiveness of treatments and make adjustments if necessary.

Active patient participation

The patient is at the center of the pain management process:

- **Open communication**: Honestly expressing pain levels and concerns to caregivers.
- **Adherence to treatment**: Follow prescriptions and recommendations to optimize results.
- **Self-management**: Use relaxation techniques, keep a pain diary to identify triggers.

Challenges and ethical considerations

1. **Opioid stigma**
   - **Fear of dependence**: May lead to under-use of opioids despite their necessity.
   - **Balanced approach**: Caregivers must weigh benefits and risks, carefully monitoring usage.

2. **Access to palliative care**
   - **Inequalities**: Some patients may have limited access to treatment due to geographical or socio-economic factors.
   - **Promoting equity**: Healthcare systems must work to make relief care accessible to all.

- Quality of life and respect for patients' wishes

Quality of life is a central concept in medicine that goes far beyond the mere absence of disease or infirmity. It encompasses the physical, mental and social well-being of the individual. In healthcare, respecting patients' wishes is essential to improving their quality of life, particularly when faced with a chronic or terminal illness. This patient-centered approach recognizes the patient's right to autonomy, dignity and active participation in decisions concerning his or her health.

Understanding patient quality of life

Quality of life is a subjective notion that varies from one individual to another. It is influenced by several factors:

1. **Physical well-being**: Effective pain and symptom management, maintenance of mobility and independence, ability to perform daily activities.

2. **Emotional well-being**: Psychological balance, absence of anxiety or depression, sense of personal accomplishment.

3. **Social relationships**: Support from family and friends, social integration, participation in community activities.

4. **Spiritual aspect**: Meaning given to life, religious or philosophical beliefs that bring comfort.

5. **Autonomy and control**: The ability to make decisions about your own life and medical care.

Respecting the patient's wishes

Respecting patients' wishes is fundamental to ethical, humanist medical practice. It is based on several principles:

1. **Autonomy**: Patients have the right to make informed decisions about their health, including refusing or accepting specific treatments.

2. **Informed consent**: Healthcare professionals must provide clear and comprehensive information on treatment options, benefits and risks, so that patients can make informed choices.

3. **Confidentiality**: Patients' personal and medical information must be protected, respecting their privacy.

4. **Dignity**: Treating patients with respect, recognizing their intrinsic value as human beings.

Practical applications in healthcare

1. **Palliative and end-of-life care**
   Palliative care aims to improve the quality of life of patients with serious illnesses by relieving pain and other symptoms. It includes psychological, social and spiritual support. Respecting patients' wishes in this context means :

   - **Listen to your preferences** regarding treatments, care settings (home, hospital, hospice) and aggressive medical interventions.
   - **Addressing advance directives**: Document the patient's wishes regarding future care, in the event of incapacity to express his/her decisions.
   - **Support the family**: Provide information and support to family members to help them understand and respect the patient's choices.

2. **Managing chronic diseases**
   Patients with chronic illnesses, such as diabetes or cardiovascular disease, often have to manage complex treatments over the long term. Respecting their wishes involves :

   - **Establish a personalized care plan**: Adapt treatments to the patient's needs and preferences.

- **Promoting therapeutic education**: helping patients to understand their illness and take charge of their health.
- **Promote autonomy**: Encourage patients to actively participate in decision-making and manage their condition on a daily basis.

3. **Communication and the therapeutic relationship**

   Open and empathetic communication between patients and healthcare professionals is essential:

   - **Active listening**: Take the time to understand the patient's concerns, values and expectations.
   - **Clear language**: Use understandable terms, avoid medical jargon.
   - **Empathy**: Recognizing and validating the patient's emotions, creating a climate of trust.

4. **Respecting cultural and spiritual differences**

   Cultural and spiritual beliefs can influence perceptions of illness and preferences for care:

   - **Cultural sensitivity**: Being aware of traditions and practices that may affect patient decisions.
   - **Adapting care**: Integrate cultural considerations into the care plan wherever possible.
   - **Working with cultural mediators**: Use interpreters or advisers to facilitate communication and mutual understanding.

Challenges and ethical considerations

1. **Complex decisions**

   Sometimes, the patient's wishes may conflict with medical recommendations or the opinions of loved ones. It is important to :

- **Navigating with delicacy**: Balancing respect for the patient's wishes with the professional obligations of beneficence and non-maleficence.
- **Engage in ethical discussion**: Involve a multidisciplinary team to explore options and implications.

2. **Patients unable to communicate**

When patients are unable to express their wishes (coma, advanced dementia), it is crucial to :

- **Refer to advance directives**: If they exist, they provide clear indications of the patient's preferences.
- **Consult legal representatives**: Family members or legal guardians can help you make decisions in line with the patient's values.

3. **Limited resources**

The constraints of the healthcare system can affect the ability to respond to the patient's wishes:

- **Transparency**: Inform the patient of possible limitations and work together to find satisfactory alternatives.
- **Advocacy**: Professionals can advocate the patient's needs to institutions to obtain the necessary resources.

The role of healthcare professionals

Physicians, nurses and other caregivers are responsible for :

- **Engage in patient-centered practice**: Putting the patient's needs and wishes at the heart of care.
- **Develop their communication skills**: Ongoing training to improve listening skills, empathy and information transmission.

- **Adopt an interdisciplinary approach**: Collaborate with other professionals (psychologists, social workers, chaplains) to address the various aspects of patient well-being.

Implications for healthcare policy

Healthcare systems must support respect for patients' wishes by :

- **Facilitating access to palliative care**: Developing specialized services to support patients at the end of life.
- **Promoting advance directives**: Raising public awareness and simplifying the process of drafting these documents.
- **Ensuring appropriate training**: Integrating ethics, communication and pain management into professional training.

- Holistic approach: physical, psychological, social and spiritual

The comprehensive approach, also known as the holistic approach, is an integrative view of the human being that considers the individual as a whole, taking into account physical, psychological, social and spiritual dimensions. This perspective recognizes that these aspects are interconnected and mutually influence a person's well-being and health. By adopting a holistic approach, health professionals, educators and social actors can better understand the complex needs of individuals and offer more effective, personalized interventions.

Physical dimension

The physical dimension concerns the body and its biological functions. It encompasses physical health, nutrition, physical activity, sleep and the management of illness or disability.

Taking care of the body is essential to maintaining good general health. This involves :

- **Balanced diet**: Providing the body with the nutrients it needs to function efficiently.
- **Regular exercise**: Improve muscular strength, flexibility, endurance and cardiovascular health.
- **Restorative sleep**: Allow the body to recover and regenerate.
- **Disease prevention**: Vaccinations, regular screening and adoption of healthy behaviors to reduce the risk of disease.

However, physical health cannot be fully understood without considering the psychological, social and spiritual influences that can affect the body.

Psychological dimension

The psychological dimension refers to mental and emotional processes, including thoughts, feelings, attitudes and beliefs. It is crucial to overall well-being, as the mind influences the body and vice versa. Key elements include:

- **Mental health**: Management of stress, anxiety, depression and other psychological disorders.
- **Self-perception**: self-esteem, self-confidence and body image.
- **Resilience**: Ability to face challenges and adapt to change.
- **Personal development**: Continuous learning, self-realization and personal fulfillment.

Emotions and thoughts can have a significant impact on physical health. For example, chronic stress can contribute to cardiovascular problems, while a positive attitude can promote healing.

Social dimension

The social dimension concerns relationships and interactions with others. Human beings are intrinsically social, and support from family, friends and the community is essential for well-being. Important aspects include:

- **Interpersonal relationships**: Quality of family, friends and professional relationships.
- **Social support**: Emotional, material and practical help received from others.
- **Community involvement**: Participation in group activities, volunteering and a sense of belonging.
- **Communication**: Ability to express needs, listen and understand others.

Social isolation or conflicting relationships can have a negative impact on mental and physical health. Conversely, a strong social network can provide crucial support in times of difficulty.

Spiritual dimension

The spiritual dimension refers to the search for meaning, purpose and connection with something greater than oneself. It is not necessarily limited to religion, but also encompasses the values, beliefs and principles that guide a person's life. The key elements are :

- **Meaning of life**: Understanding one's role and contribution to the world.
- **Personal values**: moral and ethical principles that guide our actions.
- **Spiritual practices**: Meditation, prayer, contemplation or other activities that nourish the soul.
- **Connection**: A sense of belonging to a larger reality, whether through nature, art or community.

The spiritual dimension can offer comfort, hope and a perspective that helps us through trials. It can also influence health choices and behavior.

Interconnecting dimensions

These four dimensions do not operate in isolation; they are closely interrelated and influence each other. For example:

- **Stress and physical health**: Psychological stress can weaken the immune system, making the body more vulnerable to disease.
- **Social support and mental health**: A strong social network can mitigate the effects of anxiety and depression.
- **Spirituality and resilience**: Spiritual beliefs can strengthen the ability to cope with difficult situations.
- **Physical activity and emotional well-being**: Regular exercise can improve mood and reduce depressive symptoms.

Application of the global approach

1. **In medicine and healthcare**
   Healthcare professionals who take a holistic approach assess not only physical symptoms, but also the psychological, social and spiritual factors that can affect a patient's health. This may involve:

   - **In-depth history**: Include questions about lifestyle, emotional well-being, relationships and beliefs.
   - **Personalized treatment plans**: Tailor medical interventions to the patient's overall needs and preferences.
   - **Interdisciplinary collaboration**: Work with psychologists, social workers, spiritual advisors and other specialists.

2. **In education**
   Educators can support students' overall development by :

   - **Physical health promotion**: Encourage physical activity and healthy eating.
   - **Emotional support**: Providing a safe environment for expressing emotions and developing emotional intelligence.
   - **Social development**: Fostering collaboration, mutual respect and communication skills.
   - **Spiritual awakening**: Encouraging reflection on values, meaning and purpose.

3. **At work**
   Employers can improve employee well-being by :

   - **Ergonomic design**: Preventing injuries and promoting physical health.
   - **Stress management**: Offering resources for stress management and work-life balance.
   - **Positive corporate culture**: fostering an inclusive, supportive environment.
   - **Sense of purpose**: Aligning company missions with employee values.

Advantages of the global approach

- **Improved well-being**: By addressing all aspects of life, individuals can achieve optimal health.
- **Disease prevention**: A holistic vision enables us to identify and treat risk factors before they lead to health problems.
- **Increased resilience**: People are better equipped to face challenges when they are supported on all fronts.
- **Greater satisfaction**: A balanced, meaningful life leads to greater satisfaction and fulfillment.

Challenges and considerations

- **Complexity**: Multidimensional assessment and intervention require time and resources.
- **Training**: Professionals need to be trained to recognize and address the different aspects of the holistic approach.
- **Personalization**: Every individual is unique, and solutions must be tailored to their specific needs.
- **Collaboration**: Requires coordination between different professionals and services.

Accompanying patients at the end of life

- Presence and attentive listening

Presence and attentive listening are fundamental skills that enrich our daily interactions and strengthen the quality of our relationships. They enable us to establish deep bonds, foster mutual understanding and create an environment conducive to everyone's well-being. These skills are not innate to everyone, but they can be cultivated and developed with intention and practice. This book explores the principles of presence and attentive listening, their importance in a variety of life contexts, and how we can integrate them into our daily lives.

Understanding the benevolent presence

Caring presence is the art of being fully present, physically and mentally, with an attitude of openness and compassion towards others. It involves making oneself available to others without distraction or judgment, paying sincere attention to their words, emotions and needs.

1. **Being in the present moment**: This means freeing ourselves from thoughts of the past or future to focus on the present moment. Mindfulness helps to achieve this

state, allowing us to perceive each moment with clarity and without prejudice.

2. **Adopt an attitude of openness**: Welcome the other person with benevolent curiosity, without preconceived ideas. This fosters a space where others feel safe to express themselves freely.

3. **Empathize**: Put yourself in the other person's shoes to understand their feelings and perspectives. Empathy strengthens connection and mutual trust.

The foundations of sympathetic listening

Listening goes beyond the passive hearing of spoken words. It's an active process that requires sustained attention and a sincere intention to understand the other person.

1. **Active listening**: Involve all the senses to understand the verbal and non-verbal message. This includes maintaining eye contact, observing facial expressions and gestures, and paying attention to tone of voice.

2. **Non-judgmental**: Avoid making judgments or interrupting with unsolicited advice. This creates an environment where the other person feels respected and valued.

3. **Reflective responses**: Respond appropriately by reflecting what has been said, asking open-ended questions to deepen understanding, and expressing support.

4. **Patience**: Allow others to express themselves at their own pace, without rushing or pressuring them to find immediate solutions.

The importance of presence and attentive listening

1. **Strengthening personal relationships**: Attentive listening and authentic presence strengthen emotional bonds, improve communication and promote conflict resolution.

2. **Improved mental health**: For the listener, feeling listened to and understood can reduce stress, anxiety and loneliness. For the listener, it can increase empathy and relational satisfaction.

3. **Professional effectiveness**: In the workplace, these skills improve collaboration, team motivation and customer satisfaction.

4. **Personal development**: Cultivating presence and listening enriches self-awareness, patience and the ability to live each moment to the full.

How to develop presence and good listening skills

1. **Practicing mindfulness**: Exercises such as meditation, conscious breathing or yoga can help improve concentration and awareness of the present moment.

2. **Eliminate distractions**: When interacting, put aside phones, screens and other distractions to be fully available.

3. **Develop empathy**: Reading, traveling and exposure to different cultural perspectives can enrich understanding and compassion for others.

4. **Improve communication skills**: Attend workshops or read books on non-violent communication and active listening.

5. **Self-reflection**: Take the time to reflect on your own reactions and biases to better manage them during interactions.

Practical applications in a variety of contexts

1. **Family relationships**: Promotes better understanding between family members, reduces tensions and strengthens emotional bonds.
2. **Education**: Teachers who practise good listening can better support their students, foster a positive classroom climate and encourage engagement.
3. **Healthcare**: Patient-focused healthcare professionals improve quality of care, treatment adherence and patient satisfaction.
4. **Workplace**: Managers and colleagues who actively listen can better understand challenges, stimulate innovation and create a positive corporate culture.

Challenges to overcome

1. **Time pressure**: In a fast-paced society, it can be difficult to take the time needed for attentive listening. Scheduling time for important conversations can help.
2. **Personal stress**: Personal concerns can interfere with the ability to be present for others. Taking care of one's own mental health is essential to being available for others.
3. **Unconscious biases**: Recognizing and working on your own biases can improve the quality of your listening and presence.

4. **Lack of practice**: Like any skill, presence and sympathetic listening improve with regular practice and perseverance.

Impact on society

By integrating presence and attentive listening into our daily interactions, we can :

- **Promote mutual understanding**: Reduce misunderstandings and conflicts within communities.
- **Strengthening social cohesion**: Creating stronger links between individuals, fostering a more empathetic and supportive society.
- **Promoting collective well-being**: Better communication leads to healthier environments, whether at home, at school or at work.

- Managing end-of-life events

The end of life is an inevitable stage of human existence, marked by a series of physical, psychological, social and spiritual manifestations. Effective management of these events is essential to ensure optimal quality of life for terminally ill people and to support their loved ones. A holistic, patient-centred approach helps to meet the complex and varied needs that emerge at this crucial stage.

Understanding the end of life

End-of-life is characterized by a progressive decline in vital functions, often associated with chronic or terminal illness. The focus of care shifts from cure to symptom relief, comfort and dignity. The aim is to preserve the best possible quality of life, taking into account the wishes and values of the person concerned.

Managing physical events

1. **Pain relief**
   Pain is one of the most feared symptoms at the end of life. Regular, accurate pain assessment is essential to adapt treatments. Analgesics, particularly opioids, are used to control moderate to severe pain. It is important to adjust doses to balance efficacy and side effects, while avoiding excessive sedation.

2. **Dyspnea management**
   Difficulty breathing is common and can be a source of anxiety. Treatments include:

   - **Oxygen therapy**: Administration of oxygen to improve oxygen saturation.
   - **Medication**: Low-dose opioids to reduce the sensation of dyspnea.
   - **Non-pharmacological techniques**: Patient positioning, room ventilation, use of ventilators.

3. **Controlling gastrointestinal symptoms**

   - **Nausea and vomiting**: Use of antiemetics, diet adjustment, aromatherapy.
   - **Constipation**: Laxatives, adequate hydration, adjustment of constipating medications.
   - **Anorexia and cachexia**: Respect food preferences, avoid forced feeding, nutritional supplementation if desired by patient.

4. **Managing fatigue and weakness**
   Fatigue can be profound at the end of life. It is important to :

   - **Plan activities**: Prioritize important moments for the patient.

- **Encourage rest**: Promote a calm environment for sleep.
- **Adapting the environment**: Facilitating movement and daily activities.

5. **Management of neurological disorders**
   - **Agitation and delirium**: Identification of potential causes (drugs, infections), use of sedatives if necessary, soothing environment.
   - **Convulsions**: Administration of anticonvulsants, close monitoring.

Psychological support

1. **Managing anxiety and depression**
   Feelings of anxiety, sadness or fear are common. Possible interventions include:
   - **Supportive therapy**: Interviews with a psychologist or psychiatrist.
   - **Medication**: Antidepressants or anxiolytics as required.
   - **Relaxation techniques**: meditation, deep breathing, music therapy.

2. **Emotional support**
   - **Attentive presence**: Being available to listen without judgment.
   - **Emotional validation**: Recognize the feelings expressed by the patient.
   - **Encouraging expression**: Share fears, regrets and hopes.

Social aspects

1. Involving family and friends

- **Open communication**: Facilitating dialogue between patients and their families.
- **Caregiver support**: Offering resources and respite to prevent burnout.
- **Care planning**: Include the family in decision-making, with the patient's consent.

2. Care coordination

- **Multidisciplinary team**: collaboration between doctors, nurses, social workers and psychologists.
- **Access to resources**: Referrals to home help services, hospices or support associations.

Spiritual dimension

1. Spiritual support

- **Respect for beliefs**: Take into account the patient's religious or philosophical values.
- **Access to spiritual advisors**: priests, chaplains, spiritual guides, depending on the patient's wishes.
- **Rituals and practices**: Facilitate the performance of rituals or spiritual practices.

2. Searching for meaning

- **Exploring existential questions**: Enabling patients to address profound issues about the meaning of life and death.
- **Leaving a legacy**: Helping the patient pass on memories, messages or teachings to loved ones.

Ethical and legal considerations

1. **Respecting patient autonomy**

    - **Informed consent**: Ensuring that the patient understands treatment options.
    - **Advance directives**: Encourage the drafting of directives for future care.
    - **End-of-life decisions**: Respect choices regarding the acceptance or refusal of certain treatments.

2. **Confidentiality and dignity**

    - **Protecting information**: Keeping discussions and care confidential.
    - **Respect for the individual**: Treat patients with dignity, avoiding any form of discrimination or mistreatment.

The role of healthcare professionals

1. **Effective communication**

    - **Clarity and empathy**: Explain complex situations with compassion.
    - **Active listening**: Allowing the patient and family to ask questions and express concerns.

2. **Continuing education**

    - **Palliative care skills**: learning the latest practices to improve care.
    - **Stress management**: Recognize your own limits and seek support to prevent burn-out.

Importance of the environment

1. **Patient comfort**

   - **Space planning**: cosy room, personal objects, photos.
   - **Noise and light management**: Creating a soothing atmosphere.

2. **Access to care**

   - **Home care**: Whenever possible, allow patients to remain at home.
   - **Specialized facilities**: Hospices or palliative care units offering an adapted environment.

Support after death

1. **Supporting loved ones**

   - **Bereavement**: Offering resources to help families through the grieving process.
   - **Support groups**: Connect loved ones with others who have gone through similar experiences.

2. **Commemorative rituals**

   - **Ceremonies**: Help organize funerals or memorials according to the wishes of the deceased.
   - **Tributes**: Encourage expressions of remembrance and tribute to honor the memory of the deceased.

- Respect for rituals and beliefs

Respect for rites and beliefs is a fundamental principle in a pluralistic, multicultural society. It's about recognizing and valuing the diversity of traditions, religions and philosophies of life that enrich our world. In the healthcare field, this respect is essential for providing quality, patient-centered care, and for establishing a relationship of trust between caregivers and the people they care for. Understanding and integrating people's rituals and beliefs not only helps meet their physical needs, but also supports their psychological, social and spiritual well-being.

The importance of respecting rites and beliefs

1. **Patient dignity and autonomy**
   Each individual has a unique identity, shaped by his or her culture, religion and personal convictions. Respecting a person's rites and beliefs means recognizing his or her intrinsic dignity and right to autonomy. This means considering the patient not just as a body to be cared for, but as a complete human being with values and spiritual needs that influence his or her perception of health, illness and care.

2. **Quality of care**
   Taking into account rituals and beliefs can have a direct impact on the effectiveness of treatment. For example, some patients may have dietary restrictions, fasting practices or preferences for animal or plant-based medicines. Ignoring these aspects can lead to non-adherence to treatment or unnecessary distress. By integrating these considerations, caregivers can tailor care to be both acceptable and effective for the patient.

3. **Communication and trust**
   Open communication, respectful of the patient's beliefs, helps to establish a relationship of trust. When patients

feel understood and respected, they are more inclined to share essential information about their condition, fears and expectations. This trust facilitates the patient's collaboration and commitment to his or her care.

4. **Conflict prevention**

   Failure to respect rituals and beliefs can lead to misunderstanding, tension and even conflict between patients, their families and healthcare professionals. By being sensitive to these aspects, caregivers can prevent delicate situations and ensure a serene environment for all.

Practical applications in healthcare

1. **Professional training**

   - **Cultural awareness**: Caregivers need to be trained in cultural and religious diversity to understand the practices and beliefs common in the population they serve.
   - **Intercultural communication skills**: Develop skills to communicate effectively with patients from different backgrounds, taking into account linguistic and cultural nuances.

2. **Patient needs assessment**

   - **Cultural and spiritual history**: Include questions about beliefs, religious practices and cultural preferences in the initial assessment.
   - **Personalizing care**: Adapting care plans to the patient's specific needs, for example by respecting prayer times or offering meals in line with dietary restrictions.

3. **Respect for ritual practices**

    - **Spiritual guidance**: Facilitate access to spiritual or religious advisors if the patient so wishes.
    - **Participation in rituals**: To enable rites or ceremonies to be performed whenever possible, even in a hospital environment, while ensuring the safety and respect of other patients.

4. **Managing special situations**

    - **Blood transfusions**: Some patients, for religious reasons, refuse transfusions. It's important to discuss possible alternatives and respect their decisions, while informing them of the risks.
    - **End-of-life care**: Beliefs about death and the afterlife can influence a patient's wishes regarding palliative treatment, resuscitation or rituals after death.

Challenges and solutions

1. **Language barriers**

    - **Professional interpreters**: Use qualified interpreters to avoid misunderstandings.
    - **Multilingual educational material**: Providing care information in the patient's own language.

2. **Conflicts between beliefs and medical practices**

    - **Open dialogue**: Engage in respectful discussion to understand the patient's concerns and explain medical recommendations.
    - **Seeking compromise**: Exploring solutions that respect the patient's beliefs while ensuring safe and effective care.

3. **Prejudice and stereotypes**

    - **Personal reflection**: Caregivers need to be aware of their own biases and work to overcome them.
    - **Ongoing training**: Participate in training on diversity and inclusion to improve professional practices.

The role of healthcare institutions

1. **Inclusive policies**

    - **Respect charters**: Establish policies that affirm the institution's commitment to respecting patients' rites and beliefs.
    - **Adapted protocols**: Develop procedures to manage specific requests linked to religious or cultural practices.

2. **Welcoming environment**

    - **Dedicated spaces**: Create multi-faith prayer spaces accessible to patients and families.
    - **Clear signage**: Use symbols and indications that can be understood by everyone, including those who don't speak the local language.

3. **Community involvement**

    - **Partnerships**: Collaborate with community and faith-based organizations to better understand needs and build trust with different communities.
    - **Educational events**: Organize workshops and seminars to raise staff and public awareness of cultural and religious diversity.

Ethical and legal implications

1. **Patients' rights**

    - **Freedom of religion**: Patients have the right to practice their religion and rites, as long as they do not harm others.
    - **Informed consent**: Patients' treatment decisions must be respected, even if they go against medical recommendations.

2. **Balancing respect and safety**

    - **Professional responsibility**: Caregivers must ensure the patient's safety while respecting his or her beliefs.
    - **Legal limits**: Certain practices may be restricted by law for reasons of public health or safety.

Family support

- Communication on the evolution of the patient's condition

Communication about a patient's progress is essential in the healthcare sector, for the patient, his or her family and the healthcare professionals involved. Effective communication ensures mutual understanding, builds trust and facilitates informed decision-making. It is at the heart of patient-centered care, respectful of patients' rights, needs and expectations.

Importance of communication on the evolution of the patient's condition

1. **Respecting patients' rights**
    Patients have the right to be informed about their state of health, proposed treatments, risks and possible

alternatives. This information is an essential prerequisite for informed consent, a fundamental principle of medical ethics. Transparent, honest communication enables patients to play an active role in their care.

2. **Psychological support** Being informed about the progress of your condition can help you to better manage the stress, anxiety and uncertainty associated with your illness. It enables them to prepare themselves mentally for the stages to come, mobilize their personal resources and enlist the support of their loved ones.

3. **Building trust**
Open communication strengthens the therapeutic relationship between patient and healthcare professionals. The trust thus established promotes treatment compliance, cooperation and overall patient satisfaction.

4. **Family involvement**
Relatives often play a crucial role in supporting the patient. Keeping them adequately informed enables them to better understand the situation, provide appropriate support and participate in decision-making when the patient so wishes.

Principles of effective communication

1. **Clarity and simplicity**
Use clear language, avoiding medical jargon, so that patients and their families fully understand the information conveyed. It's important to regularly check understanding and encourage questions.

2. **Empathy and respect**
Adopt a caring attitude, acknowledging the patient's emotions and concerns. Listen actively, without judgment, to create a climate of trust.

3. **Tailor-made for each patient**
Take into account individual characteristics such as age, culture, level of education and personal preferences. Adapt communication to meet the specific needs of each individual.

4. **Confidentiality**
Respect medical confidentiality by ensuring that sensitive information is only communicated to people authorized by the patient.

5. **Continuity of information**
Ensure regular communication on the evolution of the patient's condition, particularly during transitions in care (change of department, hospital discharge, etc.). This avoids information gaps and ensures consistent care.

Methods and strategies for successful communication

1. **Interview preparation**

    - **Choice of time and place**: Prefer a calm, uninterrupted environment where the patient feels at ease.
    - **Content planning**: Identify key points to be addressed, anticipate possible questions.

2. **Use of visual aids**

    - **Brochures, diagrams, images**: These can make complex information easier to understand.
    - **Digital media**: Explanatory videos, interactive applications to illustrate explanations.

3. **Communication techniques**

    - **Active listening**: Show interest, rephrase the patient's words to validate understanding.
    - **Open-ended questions**: Encourage patients to express their feelings, concerns and expectations.
    - **Feedback**: Ask the patient to summarize what he or she has understood, to ensure that the information is clear.

4. **Multidisciplinary team involvement**

    - **Coordination between professionals**: Ensure that all team members transmit consistent information.
    - **Role of nurses, psychologists, social workers**: They can provide additional support and answer specific questions.

Challenges and obstacles to effective communication

1. **Language and cultural barriers**

    - **Professional interpreters**: Use them to avoid misunderstandings.
    - **Cultural sensitivity**: Being aware of cultural differences that can influence perceptions of illness and care.

2. **Patient's emotional state**

    - **Anxiety, denial, anger**: These emotions can interfere with the reception of information.
    - **Progressive approach**: adapt the pace and content of communication to the emotional state.

3. **Complex medical information**

    - **Simplification without simplism**: Striking a balance between medical precision and patient understanding.
    - **Avoid information overload**: Provide information in stages, prioritizing essential elements.

4. **Limited time**

    - **Time management**: planning communication meetings, using time efficiently.
    - **Documentation**: Provide written material that the patient can consult at a later date.

Ethical and legal aspects

1. **Truth and transparency**

    - **Duty to inform**: The healthcare professional has a duty to provide accurate information about the patient's condition.
    - **Managing the truth**: Adapting the way things are said, while respecting the patient's right to the truth.

2. **Informed consent**

    - **Shared decision-making**: Involving the patient in therapeutic choices, after providing all the necessary information.
    - **Decision-making ability**: Assess whether the patient is able to understand and make decisions; if not, involve the legal representative.

3. Privacy

    - **Respect for medical confidentiality**: Do not divulge information without the patient's consent.
    - **Communication with relatives**: Clarify with the patient what information can be shared and with whom.

The role of information technology

1. Electronic medical records

    - **Secure information sharing**: Facilitates data transmission between professionals while preserving confidentiality.
    - **Patient access**: Some systems allow patients to consult their own files, promoting transparency.

2. Teleconsultations

    - **Continuity of communication**: maintains the link with the patient at a distance, particularly in the event of reduced mobility.
    - **Digital media**: Applications, online platforms to inform and support patients.

Training for healthcare professionals

1. Communication skills

    - **Training programs**: Integrate dedicated communication modules into medical and paramedical curricula.
    - **Practical workshops**: role-playing and simulations to develop interpersonal skills.

2. **Empathy awareness**

    o **Developing emotional intelligence**: learning to recognize and manage one's own emotions and those of the patient.
    o **Self-assessment and feedback**: Encourage reflection on one's own practice to ensure continuous improvement.

- Help with administrative formalities

Help with administrative procedures is an essential aspect of supporting individuals in their interactions with public and private institutions. Administrative procedures can often be complex, lengthy and confusing, creating obstacles for those unfamiliar with the system or facing particular difficulties. Providing appropriate support not only facilitates access to rights and services, but also promotes social inclusion and well-being.

Importance of administrative assistance

1. **Access to rights and services**

    Administrative procedures are the means by which individuals gain access to various rights and benefits, such as family allowances, housing benefit, healthcare benefits or pensions. Without a clear understanding of the procedures involved, many people risk missing out on the benefits to which they are entitled.

2. **Reducing inequalities**

    Vulnerable people, such as the elderly, people with disabilities, migrants or those with low literacy levels, are often the most affected by administrative complexity. Helping people through the administrative process helps to reduce inequalities by offering targeted support to those who need it most.

3. **Administrative efficiency**
Efficient assistance also helps to improve administrative efficiency by reducing errors, delays and incomplete applications. This facilitates the work of administrative staff and speeds up processing.

Help with administrative formalities

1. **Individual support**

    - **Social services and associations**: Many organizations offer personalized support to help individuals fill in forms, gather the necessary documents and understand procedures.

    - **Mediators and social workers**: These professionals can intervene to facilitate communication between users and administrations, solve problems and defend people's rights.

2. **Information and orientation**

    - **Information centers**: Local information points, such as Maisons de services au public (public services centers), provide information on the steps to be taken and direct users to the appropriate services.

    - **Guides and brochures**: Explanatory documents, often available in several languages, help you to understand the steps to be taken and the conditions to be met.

3. **Online help**

    - **Official websites**: Administrations offer online portals with electronic forms, tutorials and FAQs to guide users.

- **Telephone assistance**: Dedicated telephone numbers are available to help you solve problems or obtain information.

4. **Interpreting and translation services**
   For people who don't speak the local language, interpreting services can be essential for understanding administrative requirements and communicating effectively with the authorities.

Challenges faced by users

1. **Complex procedures**
   Procedures can involve multiple steps, complex forms and specific requirements, which can be discouraging.

2. **Language and cultural barriers**
   Migrants and refugees may encounter difficulties due to language or cultural differences in the way public services operate.

3. **Limited access to technology**
   With the increasing digitization of services, those who do not have access to the Internet or who are not comfortable with digital tools can be left behind.

4. **Lack of awareness of rights**
   Some people are unaware of the assistance and benefits to which they are entitled, or do not know how to apply for them.

Solutions to improve administrative support

1. **Simplified procedures**
   - **Clearer processes**: Reduce the number of forms, harmonize the documents required and simplify the language used.

- **Accessible dematerialization**: Design websites that are intuitive, compatible with mobile devices and suitable for people with disabilities.

2. **Professional training**

    - **Reception awareness**: Train administrative staff in active listening, empathy and intercultural communication.

    - **Digital skills**: Equipping social workers and mediators to help users use online tools.

3. **Strengthening community support**

    - **Volunteer networks**: Encourage volunteers to help people with their affairs.

    - **Partnerships with associations**: Working with local organizations to reach marginalized populations.

4. **Information accessibility**

    - **Multilingualism**: Offer documents and services in the languages most widely spoken by users.

    - **Varied media**: Use videos, infographics and hands-on workshops to explain the process.

Administrative assistance case studies

- **Maisons France Services**
  In France, Maisons France Services offer a one-stop shop where citizens can access a multitude of administrative services. Trained staff are on hand to help users with everything from tax returns and social security applications to identity document renewals.

- **Justice Points**
  These structures enable people to obtain free legal advice, understand their rights and be assisted in legal or administrative procedures.

- **Migrant aid associations**
  Organizations such as Cimade and France Terre d'Asile offer specific support to foreign nationals, helping them to regularize their situation and gain access to healthcare or employment.

The role of technology in administrative assistance

1. **Mobile applications**
   Dedicated applications can guide users step-by-step through the process, send reminders of deadlines or enable them to scan and send documents.

2. **Chatbots and virtual assistance**
   Chatbots can answer frequently asked questions, guide users and help them navigate administrative sites.

3. **Collaborative platforms**
   Online forums and communities enable people to share experiences, help each other and find solutions to problems.

- Presence in the final moments

Being present during the last moments of a person's life is a profoundly human and meaningful act. It represents essential support for the patient at the end of life, providing comfort, dignity and respect. This attentive, caring presence accompanies the patient in his or her final moments, ensuring that physical, emotional and spiritual needs are taken into account. Understanding the importance of this presence and knowing how to manifest it is crucial for loved ones, caregivers and all those who wish to offer meaningful accompaniment.

The importance of being present at the end of a patient's life

1. **Emotional support**
    The end of life is often a vulnerable time, marked by feelings of fear, anxiety, sadness and loneliness. The presence of a loving support person can bring immense comfort to the patient, helping them to feel less isolated and reinforcing their sense of security. The simple knowledge that someone is there, ready to listen or share a moment of silence, can ease worries and anxieties.

2. **Communication and listening** Being present also means listening attentively. Patients may feel the need to share their thoughts, memories, regrets or wishes. Open, sincere communication is the key to expressing repressed emotions and finding a degree of relief. It's important to create a space where the patient feels free to speak without fear of judgment or misunderstanding.

3. **Respecting the patient's wishes**
    Being present at the patient's side ensures that his or her wishes are respected, be they medical decisions, palliative care choices or preferences for end-of-life rituals. It reinforces the patient's dignity and autonomy right up to the last moment, honoring personal choices and deeply held values.

4. **Spiritual guidance**
    For many, the end of life is a time of spiritual or religious reflection. Presence can include support for the patient's spiritual practices, respecting their beliefs and facilitating access to necessary resources, such as a visit

from a religious representative or the provision of symbolic objects.

5. **Support for loved ones**
   Being present during the last moments of life is not only beneficial for the patient, but also for his or her family and friends. It provides a space for mutual support, enabling loved ones to share their emotions, comfort each other and face the ordeal together. It can also help alleviate the sense of helplessness one may feel when accompanying a loved one at the end of life.

How to show a benevolent presence

1. **Physical presence and attention** Being physically present, staying close to the patient, can have a profound impact. Simple gestures such as holding a hand, adjusting a pillow or offering a glass of water are evidence of attention to comfort. It's important to remain attentive to his needs without invading his personal space, respecting his signals and preferences.

2. **Active listening**
   Allowing patients to express themselves freely, without interruption, is essential. Asking open-ended questions, showing empathy and validating feelings are key elements of active listening. It's about creating an environment where the patient feels confident to share what they're feeling.

3. **Non-verbal communication**
   Sometimes words aren't necessary, or the patient may be unable to speak. Non-verbal communication, such as a smile, a kind look or simply sitting silently by their side, can convey a great deal of support and comfort.

4. **Respecting individual needs**
   Each person is unique in the way they experience the end of life. Some patients may prefer silence, others

conversation or music. It's essential to adapt to their preferences, respect their limits and not impose your own vision of things.

5. **Facilitating rituals and practices**
   Helping the patient perform spiritual or religious rituals, listening to favorite music, or looking at family photos together can bring great comfort. These moments celebrate the patient's life and strengthen emotional bonds.

6. **Coordination with the healthcare team**
   Collaborating with healthcare professionals to ensure that the patient's needs are met is crucial. This includes pain management, physical comfort and psychological support. Open communication with the care team enables us to anticipate needs and respond rapidly to changes in the patient's condition.

The challenges of presence at the end of life

1. **Managing emotions**
   Accompanying someone at the end of life can be emotionally challenging. It's normal to feel sadness, fear or helplessness. It's important to recognize your own emotions, not to repress them, and to seek support from friends, family or professionals if necessary.

2. **Communication difficulties**
   The patient may have difficulty communicating due to fatigue, pain or cognitive impairment. This requires patience, the use of alternative means of communication such as gestures, and attention to non-verbal cues.

3. **Family conflicts**
   Tensions or disagreements between family members can arise, especially in stressful situations. Open, respectful communication is the key to resolving conflicts. Sometimes, the intervention of a mediator or

professional can help re-establish a constructive dialogue.

4. **Personal limits**

   It's important to recognize your own limits as a caregiver. Taking care of yourself, taking breaks and accepting help from others are essential if you are to support your patient effectively and sustainably.

The role of healthcare professionals

1. **Multidisciplinary support**

   Doctors, nurses, psychologists, social workers and other professionals work together to offer comprehensive support to patients and their families. They provide symptom management, physical comfort and emotional support.

2. **Training and awareness**

   Healthcare professionals are trained to accompany patients at the end of life, to understand their specific needs and to provide an appropriate presence. They can also guide loved ones on how to support the patient.

3. **Supporting families**

   Caregivers play a key role in providing clear information, answering questions and supporting loved ones through this difficult period. They can also refer families to additional resources, such as support groups or home help services.

Cultural and spiritual aspects

1. **Respecting beliefs**

   Practices and beliefs concerning death vary according to culture and religion. It is essential to respect the rites, ceremonies and traditions that are important to the patient and his or her family, ensuring that they can be carried out wherever possible.

2. **Adapting care**

    Healthcare professionals need to be sensitive to cultural and spiritual needs, adapting care to suit the patient's values and wishes. This may include specific accommodations, such as the presence of a chaplain or adjusting care to respect religious practices.

After death

1. **Bereavement support**

    Being present doesn't necessarily stop at the moment of death. Offering support to loved ones in the early stages of bereavement is important. This can include attentive listening, gestures of comfort or referral to support resources.

2. **Funeral rites**

    Facilitating the performance of funeral rites in accordance with the wishes of the deceased and his or her family is a way of respecting his or her memory and enabling loved ones to begin the mourning process with peace of mind.

3. **Psychological support**

    Bereavement is a complex process that can require professional support. Referring loved ones to counselors, psychologists or discussion groups can help them through this difficult period.

Chapter 7

Technologies and Innovations in Geriatrics

E-health and telemedicine

- Using connected devices to monitor patients

The integration of digital technologies in healthcare has revolutionized the way patients are monitored and cared for. Connected devices play a key role in this transformation, offering new opportunities to improve quality of care, enhance patient engagement and optimize healthcare system resources. This paper explores in depth the use of connected devices for patient monitoring, examining their types, benefits, challenges and future prospects.

What are connected devices?

Connected devices, also known as connected objects or Internet of Things (IoT) in healthcare, are electronic devices equipped with sensors and wireless communication capabilities. They collect, transmit and sometimes analyze patient health data, enabling continuous, remote monitoring. These devices can be worn, implanted or installed in the patient's environment.

Types of connected devices for patient monitoring

1. **Wearables**

    - **Smartwatches and activity bracelets**: Measure heart rate, physical activity, sleep and other vital parameters.
    - **Continuous glucose monitors**: For diabetic patients, they monitor glucose levels and alert you to any abnormalities.
    - **Connected patches**: Skin adhesives that collect data such as body temperature, heart rate or respiration.

2. **Implantable devices**

    ◦ **Connected pacemakers**: Monitor heart function and detect arrhythmias.
    ◦ **Intelligent insulin pumps**: Automatically regulate insulin delivery according to the patient's needs.

3. **Home sensors**

    ◦ **Connected scales**: Track weight and body mass index, useful for managing heart or kidney failure.
    ◦ **Pulse oximeters**: Measure blood oxygen saturation, crucial for patients suffering from respiratory diseases.
    ◦ **Environmental monitoring systems**: Detect falls, movements or abnormalities in the living habits of elderly patients.

Benefits of using connected devices

1. **Real-time monitoring**
   Connected devices offer continuous monitoring of health parameters, enabling early detection of abnormalities and rapid intervention when needed. This reduces the risk of complications and improves clinical outcomes.

2. **Improved management of chronic diseases**
   For patients suffering from chronic diseases such as diabetes, hypertension or heart failure, these devices facilitate regular, personalized monitoring, helping to keep the disease under control and prevent hospitalization.

3. **Patient involvement and empowerment**
   Access to personal health data encourages patients to

actively participate in their own care. They can track their progress, understand the impact of their actions on their health, and adopt healthier behaviors.

4. **Reducing healthcare costs**

By reducing the number of unnecessary physical consultations and preventing hospitalizations, connected devices help optimize healthcare system resources and reduce overall expenditure.

Challenges and considerations

1. **Data protection and confidentiality**

The collection and transmission of sensitive data raises security and privacy concerns. It is essential to ensure that information is protected against unauthorized access and cyber-attacks.

2. **Data reliability and accuracy**

Accurate measurements are crucial for appropriate clinical decision-making. Devices must be clinically validated and regularly calibrated to ensure data reliability.

3. **The digital divide and accessibility**

Not all patients have equal access to digital technologies. Socio-economic disparities, lack of digital skills or lack of network coverage can limit the use of these devices.

4. **Integration with existing healthcare systems**

To be fully effective, connected devices need to be compatible with electronic medical records and healthcare facilities' IT systems. This requires interoperability standards and collaboration between industry players.

Use cases

1. **Cardiovascular disease monitoring**
   Devices can detect abnormal heart rhythms, monitor blood pressure and alert to early signs of heart attack or stroke.

2. **Diabetes management**
   Continuous glucose sensors and connected insulin pumps enable more precise blood glucose management, reducing the risk of hyperglycemia or hypoglycemia.

3. **Monitoring elderly patients**
   Motion sensors and alert systems can detect falls or changes in lifestyle, enabling rapid intervention and preventing deterioration in health.

4. **Rehabilitation monitoring**
   Devices can measure the physical progress of patients in rehabilitation, provide real-time feedback and adapt exercise programs accordingly.

Impact on the healthcare system

1. **Improved clinical decision-making**
   Access to accurate, up-to-date data enables healthcare professionals to make informed decisions, adjust treatments and personalize care according to individual needs.

2. **Reduced hospitalization**
   Proactive monitoring can detect problems before they require hospitalization, improving patients' quality of life and reducing the burden on healthcare facilities.

3. **Personalized care**
   The data collected enables us to better understand patients' health patterns, leading to more targeted and effective interventions.

The role of healthcare professionals

1. **Interpreting data**
   Doctors and nurses need to be trained to analyze the information provided by connected devices, identify trends and react appropriately.

2. **Communication with patients**
   Good communication is essential to explain to patients the importance of follow-up, how to use the devices and interpret the results.

3. **Adapting clinical practices**
   Integrating connected devices requires adaptation of clinical processes, including data flow management and coordination with other healthcare professionals.

Future prospects

1. **Artificial intelligence and predictive analysis**
   The use of AI can help analyze large amounts of data, identify complex patterns and predict health events, enabling even earlier intervention.

2. **Technological innovations**
   The development of new sensors, miniaturized devices and non-invasive technologies will continue to expand monitoring possibilities.

3. **Regulations and standards**
   Clear regulatory frameworks are needed to ensure the safety, efficiency and data protection associated with the use of connected devices.

- Advantages and limitations of remote monitoring

Telesurveillance, also known as telemonitoring, is the use of information and communication technologies to remotely monitor a patient's state of health. It enables healthcare professionals to monitor patients in real time, without requiring their physical presence. This innovative approach offers many advantages, but also presents certain limitations that are important to consider for effective and ethical use.

Benefits of remote monitoring

1. **Improving access to care**

   - **Reduced travel** : Patients, especially those living in rural or remote areas, can access healthcare services without having to travel, which is particularly beneficial for people with reduced mobility.
   - **Increased availability of healthcare professionals**: Telemonitoring enables doctors to monitor a greater number of patients, optimizing their time and resources.

2. **Ongoing, personalized follow-up**

   - **Early detection of complications**: Real-time monitoring of vital signs and health parameters makes it possible to quickly identify abnormalities and intervene before the situation worsens.
   - **Personalized care**: the data collected enables treatments to be tailored to the specific needs of each patient, improving the effectiveness of interventions.

3. **Improving patients' quality of life**

   - **Greater autonomy**: Patients can manage their health from home, enhancing their independence and comfort.

- **Reduced stress and anxiety**: Knowing that their state of health is constantly monitored can reassure patients and their loved ones.

4. **Optimizing healthcare system resources**

    - **Reduced hospitalization**: By preventing complications, remote monitoring helps reduce the number of hospitalizations and the length of hospital stays.

    - **Cost-effectiveness**: fewer physical consultations and hospitalizations mean savings for the healthcare system.

5. **Promoting patient involvement**

    - **Empowerment**: Patients become involved in their own health, which can improve compliance and encourage healthier behaviors.

    - **Health education**: Access to personal health data helps patients better understand their condition.

Limits of remote monitoring

1. **Privacy and data security issues**

    - **Protecting sensitive information**: The transmission and storage of healthcare data raises confidentiality concerns. Robust cybersecurity measures are needed to prevent data breaches.

    - **Regulatory compliance**: healthcare professionals and service providers must comply with data protection laws, such as the General Data Protection Regulation (GDPR) in Europe.

2. **Technological dependence**

    - **Device reliability**: Equipment malfunctions or failures can compromise patient monitoring and safety.
    - **Technological obsolescence**: Technologies evolve rapidly, making devices quickly outdated and requiring frequent updating or replacement.

3. **Unequal access**

    - **Digital divide**: Not all patients have access to a reliable Internet connection or the digital skills needed to use remote monitoring devices.
    - **Patient costs**: The acquisition and maintenance of equipment can represent a significant cost for some patients, limiting accessibility.

4. **Patient-healthcare professional relations**

    - **Reduced human interaction**: Fewer face-to-face consultations can affect the quality of the relationship between patient and healthcare professional, which in turn can influence the effectiveness of care.
    - **Risk of information overload**: An influx of data can overwhelm healthcare professionals, making it difficult to sort out the relevant information.

5. **Clinical limits**

    - **Reliability of remote measurements**: Some of the data collected may be less accurate than those obtained in a clinical setting, which can affect medical decisions.

- **Not suitable for all pathologies**: Telemonitoring is not always appropriate for certain patients or medical conditions requiring direct physical assessment.

6. Legal and ethical aspects

- **Medical liability**: Questions of liability in the event of misinterpretation of data or delay in intervention can be complex.

- **Informed consent**: It is essential that patients understand the implications of telemonitoring and give their informed consent.

Outlook and recommendations

To maximize the benefits of remote monitoring while mitigating its limitations, several actions can be considered:

- **Strengthening data security**: Implementing advanced security protocols and ensuring compliance with current regulations to protect patient confidentiality.

- **Training for patients and professionals**: Provide training to improve patients' digital skills and help healthcare professionals manage the data they collect effectively.

- **Universal accessibility**: Develop solutions to reduce the digital divide, in particular by offering adapted devices and facilitating access to a reliable Internet connection.

- **Hybrid care integration**: Combine telemonitoring with face-to-face consultations to maintain a strong relationship between patient and healthcare professional.

- **Ongoing evaluation**: Conduct research and studies to assess the effectiveness of telemonitoring in different clinical contexts and adjust practices accordingly.

- Impact on the role of the caregiver

The caregiver occupies a central position in the healthcare system, often being at the forefront of direct patient care. Recent developments in the healthcare field, whether technological, organizational or ethical, are having a significant impact on the role of the caregiver. These changes require constant adaptation to meet the complex and varied needs of patients, while complying with current regulations.

Expanded skills and responsibilities

1. **Holistic approach to care**

    - **Comprehensive patient care**: The caregiver is now encouraged to consider not only the patient's physical needs, but also their psychological, social and spiritual dimensions. This holistic approach requires a thorough understanding of each patient's individuality.
    - **Participating in needs assessment**: Working closely with nurses and other members of the care team, the caregiver contributes to the assessment of the patient's needs, providing valuable information thanks to his or her proximity to the patient.

2. **A stronger role in communication**
    - **Presence and attentive listening**: The caregiver plays a key role in the emotional support of patients, offering attentive listening and being present during difficult moments.
    - **Mediating with the family**: He can act as a link between the patient, his family and the medical team, facilitating communication and helping to clarify information.

3. **Health technology management**
    - **Use of connected devices**: With the introduction of telemonitoring and connected medical devices, caregivers need to acquire technological skills to assist patients in using these tools.
    - **Ongoing training**: The need to keep abreast of new technologies and associated protocols has become essential if we are to remain effective and relevant in our role.

Adapting to new care practices

1. **Infection prevention and hygiene**
    - **Mastery of hygiene techniques**: The caregiver is directly involved in the application of disinfection and sterilization protocols, as well as in the appropriate use of personal protective equipment (PPE).
    - **Patient education**: Participates in patient education on good hygiene practices, contributing to the prevention of nosocomial infections.

2. **Waste management and respect for the environment**

- **Waste classification and disposal**: A thorough knowledge of the different waste categories and safe disposal procedures is necessary to ensure safety and regulatory compliance.
- **Ecological awareness**: The caregiver can play a role in promoting ecological practices within the healthcare establishment.

3. **End-of-life care**

- **Accompanying patients at the end of life**: The caregiver is often present during the last moments, offering emotional support and ensuring the patient's comfort.
- **Respect for rites and beliefs**: We must be attentive to the wishes of patients and their families regarding religious or cultural rites, ensuring a respectful and dignified environment.

Occupational risk prevention

1. **Prevention of musculoskeletal disorders (MSD)**

    - **Application of ergonomic principles**: By adopting appropriate postures and using equipment correctly, caregivers protect their physical health.
    - **Gesture and posture training**: Regular training enables us to maintain a high level of competence in handling patients and loads.

2. **Stress management and well-being at work**

    - **Developing stress management skills**: Faced with sometimes trying situations, caregivers need to learn how to manage stress to preserve their mental health.

- **Institutional support**: Healthcare establishments have a role to play in providing resources and a favorable working environment.

Compliance with regulations and professional standards

1. **Compliance with protocols and procedures**

   - **Regular updating of knowledge**: Health regulations are constantly evolving, and caregivers need to keep abreast of changes to ensure compliant practice.
   - **Attendance at mandatory training courses**: Certain training courses, such as those on hygiene or waste management, are essential for maintaining legal compliance.

2. **Ethics and confidentiality**

   - **Respect for professional secrecy**: caregivers are required to maintain the confidentiality of patient information.
   - **Ethical approach to care**: Act with integrity, respect and compassion, taking into account the rights and dignity of each patient.

Continuous professional development

1. **Training and specialization**

   - **Access to further training**: To meet the changing needs of the healthcare sector, caregivers can specialize in areas such as geriatrics, pediatrics or palliative care.
   - **Career development**: Opportunities for advancement, such as becoming a gerontological care assistant or referral caregiver, are possible with appropriate training.

2. **Multidisciplinary teamwork**

    - **Interprofessional collaboration**: The caregiver works closely with nurses, doctors, physiotherapists and other professionals, contributing to the overall care of the patient.
    - **Effective communication**: Sharing relevant information and participating in team meetings are essential for optimal care coordination.

Impact of technology on the role of the caregiver

1. **Digitizing care**

    - **Use of healthcare software**: Mastery of IT tools for patient data entry, care planning and internal communication has become indispensable.
    - **Teleconsultation and telemonitoring**: The caregiver may be called upon to assist the patient during teleconsultations, ensuring that the devices are working properly and supporting the patient.

2. **Artificial intelligence and automation**

    - **Adapting to new technologies**: With the introduction of assistive robots or AI applications, caregivers must learn to integrate these tools into their daily practice.
    - **Maintaining the human aspect of care**: Despite increasing automation, the caregiver's role as a human link remains essential to the patient's well-being.

Technical Aids and Home Automation

- Presentation of autonomy-enhancing tools (smart beds, motion sensors)

Autonomy is a crucial issue for the elderly, the disabled and convalescing patients. Modern technologies now offer innovative solutions to improve their quality of life and independence on a daily basis. Among these solutions, intelligent beds and motion sensors play a key role. These devices, integrated into domestic or institutional environments, not only facilitate daily activities, but also ensure the safety and well-being of users. The aim of this talk is to present these tools, their functionalities, their advantages and their impact on the autonomy of the people concerned.

I. Smart beds

1. **Definition and features**

   Smart beds are devices equipped with advanced technologies to offer optimal comfort, monitor the user's health and facilitate care. They integrate sensors, actuators and communication systems to interact with the user and healthcare professionals.

2. **Main features**

   - **Automatic position adjustment**: Tilt the mattress to facilitate breathing, digestion or blood circulation.
   - **Vital signs monitoring**: integrated sensors to measure heart rate, respiration and body temperature.
   - **Motion detection**: Identification of nocturnal movements to analyze sleep quality.
   - **Anomaly alerts**: Notifications sent to caregivers or healthcare professionals in the event of a fall or abnormal vital parameters.

- **Connectivity**: Integration with mobile applications or home automation systems for remote control.

3. **User benefits**

    - **Personalized comfort**: adapt the bed to the user's preferences for better rest.
    - **Increased safety**: Continuous monitoring to prevent domestic accidents.
    - **Enhanced autonomy**: the bed can be controlled without assistance, using simple interfaces or voice commands.
    - **Health monitoring**: data collection for more precise medical monitoring.

4. **Practical applications**

    - **Home care**: Enabling frail people to remain safely at home.
    - **Healthcare facilities**: Facilitates the work of nursing staff and improves patient comfort.
    - **Hospitality**: Offering high-end comfort to customers, with customization options.

II. Motion sensors

1. **Definition and types of sensor**

    Motion sensors are electronic devices that detect movement in a given space. They use various technologies such as infrared, ultrasound, radar or optical cameras.

2. Main features

- **Presence detection**: Identification of the presence of a person in a room.
- **Movement tracking**: Analysis of movements to detect patterns or anomalies.
- **Fall detection** : Systems capable of recognizing a fall and immediately alerting emergency services.
- **Home automation integration**: automatic control of lighting, heating and appliances based on presence.

3. User benefits

- **Enhanced safety**: Discreet surveillance reduces the risk of domestic accidents.
- **Preserved autonomy**: users can move around freely without the constant intervention of a third party.
- **Improved comfort**: domestic equipment automatically adapts to the user's needs.
- **Peace of mind for loved ones**: Families can be informed in real time if a problem arises.

4. Practical applications

- **Connected homes**: Improving comfort and security in the home.
- **Retirement homes and EHPAD**: Monitoring residents to prevent incidents.
- **Hospitals**: Help in monitoring patients at risk of falling or running away.
- **Public spaces**: energy-saving lighting and heating management.

III Impact on user autonomy

1. **Strengthening independence**
   - **Self-managed needs**: users can adjust their environment without assistance.
   - **Reduced dependency**: less need for the constant presence of a caregiver.

2. **Improved quality of life**
   - **Increased comfort**: technologies adapt to individual preferences.
   - **Safety**: Accident prevention and rapid response to emergencies.
   - **Self-confidence**: Feeling of control over one's environment and health.

3. **Social interaction**
   - **Facilitated communication**: Devices can include features for keeping in touch with loved ones.
   - **Active participation**: Users are encouraged to get involved in managing their health.

IV. Considerations and challenges

1. **Confidentiality and data protection**
   - **Management of personal information**: Importance of securing collected data.
   - **Legal compliance**: Compliance with regulations such as the RGPD.

2. **Technological acceptance**
   - **Barriers to adoption**: Resistance to change or difficulty of use for some people.

- **Training and support**: We need to help users get to grips with the technologies.

3. **Cost and accessibility**
   - **Initial investment**: Devices can be expensive.
   - **Inequalities of access**: Risk of widening the gap between populations.

4. **Reliability and maintenance**
   - **Faults and malfunctions** : Potential impact on user safety.
   - **Updates** : Need to keep systems up to date to ensure their effectiveness.

V. Future prospects

1. **Integrating artificial intelligence**
   - **Advanced personalization**: Automatic adaptation to changing user needs and habits.
   - **Predictive analysis**: Anticipating risks and future needs.

2. **Development of norms and standards**
   - **Interoperability**: Facilitating communication between different devices and platforms.
   - **Enhanced security**: protocols in place to protect data.

3. **Greater accessibility**
   - **Democratization of technologies**: cost reduction through innovation and mass production.
   - **Assistance programs**: Subsidies or insurance to help purchase devices.

- Training in the use of modern equipment

Rapidly evolving technologies have led to the integration of modern equipment in many sectors, such as healthcare, industry, education and services. Whether it's advanced medical devices, automated industrial machinery or innovative digital tools, this equipment offers considerable advantages in terms of efficiency, precision and productivity. However, to exploit the full potential of these technologies, proper training in their use is essential. This training enables professionals to master modern tools, improve the quality of their work and ensure their own safety as well as that of others.

I. The importance of training in modern equipment

1. **Optimizing efficiency and productivity**

   Mastering modern equipment enables users to maximize their efficiency. Proper training ensures that employees understand all tool functionalities, reducing the time needed to complete tasks and minimizing errors.

2. **User and patient safety**

   In sectors such as healthcare or industry, misuse of equipment can lead to safety risks. Training ensures that users are familiar with safety protocols, emergency procedures and best practices to avoid accidents.

3. **Improved quality of service and care**

   Competent use of modern equipment translates into better quality services. In the healthcare sector, for example, this can lead to more accurate diagnoses and more effective care.

4. **Adapting to technological change**

   Technologies are constantly evolving. Ongoing training enables professionals to stay up to date, quickly adopt new working methods and maintain a competitive edge.

II. Types of modern equipment requiring training

1. Medical equipment

- **Medical imaging devices**: MRIs, scanners, ultrasound scanners.
- **Connected devices**: vital sign monitors, intelligent infusion pumps.
- **Surgical robots**: systems to assist minimally invasive surgery.
- **Medical software**: computerized patient records, telemedicine tools.

2. Automated industrial machines

- **Industrial robots**: articulated arms for assembly, welding and painting.
- **3D printers**: additive manufacturing for prototyping or production.
- **Numerical control systems**: Computer-controlled machine tools.

3. Digital tools and software

- **Integrated management software**: ERP, CRM for resource and customer relationship management.
- **Virtual and augmented reality applications**: training, design, maintenance.
- **Collaborative platforms**: tools for remote working and project management.

4. Information and communication technologies

- **Unified communications systems**: integrating voice, video and data.
- **Cyber-security**: Tools and protocols to protect sensitive information.

III. Training methods for the use of modern equipment

1. **Face-to-face training**

    - **Hands-on workshops**: Interactive sessions with experienced trainers.
    - **Live demonstrations**: Presentation of equipment in real-life situations.

2. **Online training (e-learning)**

    - **Interactive modules**: Online courses with videos, quizzes and assessments.
    - **Webinars**: Live sessions with the opportunity to ask questions.

3. **Blended learning**

    - **Combination of methods**: Alternating online and face-to-face courses for optimum flexibility.

4. **On-the-job training**

    - **Mentoring**: Support from experienced colleagues.
    - **On-the-job training**: Supervised learning in real-life situations.

5. **Using virtual and augmented reality**

    - **Immersive simulations**: virtual environments for risk-free practice.
    - **Pedagogical applications**: Interactive scenarios to reinforce learning.

IV. Training challenges and solutions

1. Resistance to change

- **Challenge**: Employees can be reluctant to adopt new technologies.
- **Solution**: Involve staff from the outset, communicate the benefits and offer ongoing support.

2. Training costs

- **Challenge**: Training can be a major investment.
- **Solution**: Use free or low-cost online resources, benefit from grants or partnerships with educational institutions.

3. Diversity of skill levels

- **Challenge**: Employees have varying levels of familiarity with technology.
- **Solution**: Customize training programs, offering basic and advanced modules.

4. Rapidly evolving technologies

- **Challenge**: Equipment and software can quickly become obsolete.
- **Solution**: Establish a culture of continuous learning, encourage technology watch.

V. The role of employers and training organizations

1. Employers' responsibilities

- **Investment in training**: Allocate resources to train staff.
- **Encouraging further training**: Valuing learning and recognizing acquired skills.

- **Creating a favorable environment**: Providing the time and tools needed for training.

2. **Contributions from training organizations**

    - **Designing adapted programs**: Developing training programs in line with market needs.
    - **Working with companies**: Understanding the specificities of the sector and adapting content.
    - **Pedagogical innovation**: Using the latest teaching methods to maximize effectiveness.

VI. Training benefits for professionals and organizations

1. **For professionals**

    - **Skills development**: Acquisition of new skills that can be put to good use in the job market.
    - **Career development**: Better prospects for advancement and professional mobility.
    - **Personal satisfaction**: A sense of accomplishment and self-confidence.

2. **For organizations**

    - **Increased competitiveness**: ability to innovate and adapt to market changes.
    - **Improved quality**: better quality products and services thanks to optimal use of equipment.
    - **Employee loyalty**: Trained and valued staff are more committed and less likely to leave the company.

- Integrating technology into daily care

The rapid evolution of information and communication technologies has profoundly transformed the healthcare sector. The integration of technologies into everyday care has become an inescapable reality, offering new opportunities to improve the quality of care, the efficiency of healthcare services and the well-being of patients. From connected medical devices and mobile health apps to artificial intelligence and telemedicine, technological innovations are redefining the way care is delivered and received. This article explores the different facets of this integration, its benefits, challenges and prospects for the future.

I. Technologies integrated into daily care

1. Connected medical devices

- **Connected health devices (IoMT)**: smartwatches, activity wristbands, continuous glucose sensors, connected blood pressure monitors.
- **Advanced medical equipment**: intelligent infusion pumps, sensor-equipped medical beds, connected pacemakers.

2. Mobile health applications (mHealth)

- **Chronic disease management**: applications for monitoring diabetes, hypertension and asthma.
- **Wellness and prevention**: Tools for monitoring physical activity, diet and sleep.

3. Telemedicine and teleconsultation

- **Remote consultations**: Videoconferences between patients and healthcare professionals.
- **Telemonitoring**: remote monitoring of health parameters for patients at home.

4. **Electronic medical records (EMR)**
    - **Centralized information**: Secure access to patient medical data by different healthcare professionals.
    - **Information sharing**: Facilitating care coordination between the various parties involved

5. **Artificial intelligence (AI) and machine learning**
    - **Diagnostic support**: AI tools for medical image analysis and early disease detection.
    - **Personalized treatment**: Algorithms to adapt therapies to individual patient characteristics.

6. **Medical robotics**
    - **Surgical robots**: Assistance during surgery for greater precision.
    - **Assistive robots:** mobility assistance for patients, support with daily tasks.

II. Benefits of integrating technology into care

1. **Improving the quality of care**
    - **Diagnostic precision**: Technological tools enable more precise and earlier detection of diseases.
    - **Personalized treatment**: Adapting care to the specific needs of each patient.

2. **Operational efficiency**
    - **Process optimization**: Reduce time spent on administrative tasks through automation.
    - **Resource management**: better allocation of personnel and equipment.

3. **Accessibility and continuity of care**
    - **Reducing geographical barriers**: Telemedicine makes it possible to reach patients in remote areas.
    - **Real-time monitoring**: Connected devices provide continuous monitoring of health status.

4. **Engaging and empowering patients**
    - **Active participation**: Patients are encouraged to manage their health through apps and connected devices.
    - **Health education**: Access to information and resources to better understand their condition.

5. **Reduced healthcare costs**
    - **Preventing complications**: Regular monitoring to avoid unnecessary hospitalization.
    - **Treatment effectiveness**: Better match between care provided and actual needs.

III. Technology integration challenges and considerations

1. **Data security and confidentiality**
    - **Protecting sensitive information**: Risks of cyber-attacks and data breaches.
    - **Regulatory compliance**: Compliance with laws such as the RGPD for the management of personal data.

2. **Unequal access**
    - **Digital divide**: Differences in access to technologies between populations.
    - **Digital skills**: Patients and professionals need to master technological tools.

3. **System interoperability**
   - **Device compatibility** : Difficulties integrating different systems and platforms.
   - **Standardization**: the need for common standards to facilitate information exchange.

4. **Training for healthcare professionals**
   - **Acquiring new skills**: the need for ongoing training to adapt to emerging technologies.
   - **Acceptance of change**: Possible resistance to adopting new working methods.

5. **Ethical aspects**
   - **The patient-caregiver relationship**: Risk of dehumanization of care with increased use of technology.
   - **Automated decisions**: Questioning liability in the event of an AI system error.

IV. Successful technology integration: best practices

1. **Patient-centered approach**
   - **Co-designing solutions**: Involving patients in the development of tools to meet their real needs.
   - **Universal accessibility**: Designing inclusive technologies for all users.

2. **Training and support for professionals**
   - **Training programs**: Offering training tailored to mastering new technologies.
   - **Institutional support**: Encouraging a culture of innovation within healthcare establishments.

3. **Enhanced system security**
   - **Implementation of security protocols**: data encryption, strong authentication.
   - **Regular audits**: Checking system compliance and robustness.

4. **Interdisciplinary collaboration**
   - **Teamwork**: Involve IT specialists, healthcare professionals, patients and managers.
   - **Knowledge sharing**: exchanges between different players to optimize the use of technologies.

5. **Assessment and continuous improvement**
   - **Performance monitoring**: Measure the impact of technologies on care and adjust accordingly.
   - **User feedback**: Gather feedback from patients and professionals to improve tools.

V. Future prospects

1. **Artificial intelligence and predictive medicine**
   - **Big data analysis**: Using large datasets to identify trends and predict health events.
   - **Personalized therapies**: Development of customized treatments based on the patient's genetic profile.

2. **Virtual and augmented reality**
   - **Medical training**: used to simulate surgical procedures.
   - **Rehabilitation**: Interactive programs to help patients recover their motor functions.

3. **3D printing in medicine**

    - **Made-to-measure prostheses**: manufacture of devices adapted to specific patient needs.
    - **Bioprinting**: prospects for the creation of organic tissue for transplants.

4. **Telesurgery and medical robots**

    - **Remote operations**: surgeons can operate on patients located in other regions.
    - **Robotic assistance**: greater precision and reduced operating risks.

5. **Blockchain for healthcare**

    - **Data security**: Use of blockchain technology to guarantee the integrity and confidentiality of medical information.
    - **Consent management**: Make it easier for patients to control access to their data.

Mobile Applications and Tracking Software

- Care management and patient records software

In today's increasingly digitized healthcare environment, care management and patient records software play a central role in improving the quality of care, operational efficiency and coordination between different healthcare players. These technological tools make it possible to centralize medical information, facilitate communication between professionals and offer patients more personalized and secure care. This article explores the different facets of care and patient record management software, their functionalities, benefits, associated challenges and future prospects.

I. Definition and importance of patient record and care management software

1. **Care management software**

   Care management software are computer applications designed to support healthcare professionals in the organization, planning and coordination of patient care. They encompass a range of tools designed to optimize clinical, administrative and financial processes within healthcare establishments.

2. **Computerized patient records (CPR)**

   The computerized patient record is a digital version of the traditional medical record. It centralizes all patient information, such as medical history, diagnoses, treatments, test results and notes from healthcare professionals. The CIO facilitates rapid, secure access to data essential to informed decision-making.

3. **Importance in the healthcare system**

   - **Improved quality of care**: By providing instant access to up-to-date patient information, software contributes to better care.
   - **Operational efficiency**: Reduced time spent on administrative tasks, enabling professionals to concentrate on care.
   - **Care coordination**: Facilitating communication between the various parties involved, avoiding redundancies and errors.
   - **Data security** : Protect sensitive information with advanced security protocols.

II. Types of care and patient record management software

1. **Hospital information systems (HIS)**

   - Integrate various functionalities to manage all the activities of a healthcare facility.
   - Includes modules for administrative, financial, logistical and clinical management.

2. **Computerized patient records (DPI)**

   - Centralize patient medical data.
   - Enable information to be shared securely between authorized professionals.

3. **Clinical Decision Support Systems (CDSS)**

   - Provide alerts, reminders and recommendations based on patient data.
   - Help with drug prescription, pointing out potential interactions.

4. **Practice management software**

   - Designed for private practices, they manage appointments, billing and patient files.
   - Facilitate patient relations via messaging and appointment reminder functionalities.

5. **Patient portals**

   - Online platforms enabling patients to access their health information.
   - Offer services such as making appointments, consulting test results and communicating with professionals.

6. **Telehealth systems**

    - Integrate functions for teleconsultation, remote monitoring and telediagnosis.
    - Facilitate access to care for patients living far away or with reduced mobility.

III. Key features of care management and patient records software

1. **Patient data management**

    - **Collection and storage**: Secure storage of medical information.
    - **Real-time** updates: Instant data updates with every interaction.

2. **Appointment scheduling and management**

    - **Integrated calendar**: Manage the availability of professionals and rooms.
    - **Automated reminders**: patient notifications to reduce absences.

3. **Clinical documentation**

    - **Notes and observations**: Structured or free input of clinical information.
    - **Protocols and forms**: Templates for standardizing data collection.

4. **Prescription management**

    - **Electronic prescriptions**: digital prescribing and transmission to pharmacies.
    - **Check for interactions**: Drug risk alerts.

5. **Billing and financial management**

    - **Payment processing**: Managing transactions with patients and insurers.
    - **Insurance management**: checking coverage and reimbursements.

6. **Communication and collaboration**

    - **Secure messaging**: information exchange between professionals.
    - **Document sharing** : Secure transmission of reports and medical images.

7. **Reports and analyses**

    - **Dashboards**: Visualize key performance indicators.
    - **Statistical analysis**: Support for research and practice improvement.

8. **Safety and compliance**

    - **Access control**: Manage authorizations to protect sensitive data.
    - **Audit and traceability**: Recording actions to ensure transparency.

IV. Advantages of care and patient record management software

1. **Improving the quality of care**

    - **Reduced medical errors**: thanks to improved availability of information.
    - **Informed decision-making**: Access to comprehensive data for accurate assessment.

2. **Increased operating efficiency**
    - **Task automation**: less paperwork, more time for patients.
    - **Optimized workflows**: Standardized processes for better coordination.

3. **Patient engagement**
    - **Active participation**: Patients can track their health and book appointments online.
    - **Improved communication**: better interaction between patients and professionals.

4. **Cost management**
    - **Reduced costs**: less duplication of tests, efficient management of resources.
    - **Accurate invoicing**: fewer errors in financial transactions.

5. **Regulatory compliance**
    - **Compliance with standards**: Helps comply with data protection laws, such as the RGPD.
    - **Proper documentation**: Facilitates audits and certifications.

V. Challenges and considerations in the use of care management software and patient records

1. **Data security and confidentiality**
    - **Risks of cyber-attacks**: need for robust measures to protect sensitive information.
    - **Legal compliance**: Compliance with regulations on the protection of personal data.

2. **Interoperability**

    - **Systems integration**: Difficulties in connecting different software and platforms.
    - **Norms and standards**: the need to adopt common protocols for information exchange.

3. **User adoption**

    - **Resistance to change**: Some professionals may be reluctant to adopt new tools.
    - **Training required**: Need to invest in training to ensure effective use.

4. **Costs and resources**

    - **Initial investment**: Software acquisition and installation costs.
    - **Maintenance and updates** : Recurring costs to ensure smooth operation.

5. **Data quality**

    - **Accuracy and completeness**: Risks associated with incorrect or incomplete data entry.
    - **Duplicate management**: Procedures to avoid multiple registrations.

VI. Regulations and legal framework

1. **Personal data protection**

    - **General Data Protection Regulation (GDPR)**: European framework for the protection of personal data.
    - **Obligations of professionals**: Informed consent, right to be forgotten, notification of violations.

2. **Software certification**

    - **Approval by the authorities**: Some software must be certified to guarantee compliance.
    - **ISO standards**: Adoption of international standards for quality and safety.

3. **Interoperability and standards**

    - **HL7, DICOM**: Protocols for medical data exchange.
    - **National initiatives**: programs to promote interoperability at national level.

VII. Future prospects

1. **Integrating artificial intelligence**

    - **Predictive analytics**: using algorithms to anticipate health risks.
    - **Virtual assistant**: Clinical documentation and decision-making support.

2. **Mobility and accessibility**

    - **Mobile applications**: Access data from mobile devices for greater flexibility.
    - **Integrated teleconsultation**: Integration of telemedicine services into management software.

3. **Patient at the center of the system**

    - **Enhanced patient portals**: more interactivity and information available to patients.
    - **Community involvement**: Tools to encourage patients to participate in their own health.

4. **Blockchain and security**

    ○ **Enhanced traceability**: use of blockchain for transparent data management.
    ○ **Secure sharing**: facilitate data exchange while guaranteeing confidentiality.

- Applications for cognitive stimulation

Cognitive stimulation is a set of activities and exercises designed to maintain or improve cognitive functions such as memory, attention, language, perception and executive functions. With the aging of the population and the increase in cognitive disorders such as Alzheimer's disease, digital applications have become invaluable tools for promoting brain health. These applications offer a variety of exercises, adapted to individual needs, and can be used at home or in an institution. This article presents the different cognitive stimulation applications, their functionalities and benefits, as well as the considerations to be taken into account when using them.

I. What is cognitive stimulation?

1. **Definition**

    Cognitive stimulation aims to stimulate and strengthen mental capacities through structured activities. It is based on cerebral plasticity, i.e. the brain's ability to reorganize itself in response to new experiences or learning.

2. **Objectives**

    ○ **Maintain cognitive functions**: prevent age-related decline or neurodegenerative diseases.
    ○ **Improve performance**: Strengthen specific abilities such as memory or attention.

- **Promote well-being**: Reduce anxiety, improve mood and self-confidence.

II. Types of applications for cognitive stimulation

1. **Brain game applications**

   - **Lumosity**: Offers games based on memory, attention, cognitive flexibility and problem-solving.
   - **Elevate**: Targets skills such as reading, writing, mathematics and listening comprehension.
   - **Peak**: Offers personalized exercises based on the user's objectives, with progress tracking.

2. **Memory and learning applications**

   - **NeuroNation**: Focuses on working memory, concentration and intelligence.
   - **CogniFit**: Evaluates the user's cognitive profile and suggests appropriate exercises.

3. **Applications for cognitive disorders**

   - **Amuse**: Designed for people with Alzheimer's disease or dementia, with specially adapted activities.
   - **HappyNeuron Pro**: Designed for healthcare professionals for the cognitive rehabilitation of patients.

4. **Virtual and augmented reality applications**

   - **MindMaze**: virtual reality for cognitive and motor rehabilitation.
   - **Memoride**: Allows users to pedal a stationary bike while exploring virtual environments, stimulating memory and motivation.

5. **Meditation and mindfulness applications**

    - **Headspace**: Helps improve concentration and reduce stress through guided meditation exercises.
    - **Calm**: Offers programs for relaxation, sleep and anxiety management.

III. Common features of cognitive stimulation applications

1. **Personalization**

    - **Adaptation to user profile**: Adjustment of difficulty level according to performance.
    - **Choice of areas to work on**: Selection of specific cognitive functions to be trained.

2. **Progress monitoring**

    - **Statistics and reports**: Visualize improvements over time.
    - **Goals and rewards**: Motivation through daily challenges and encouragement.

3. **Interactivity**

    - **Immediate feedback**: Instant information on correct or incorrect answers.
    - **Fun interface**: Attractive graphics and engaging games to maintain interest.

4. **Accessibility**

    - **Multi-platform compatibility**: Available on smartphones, tablets and computers.
    - **Ease of use**: Intuitive interfaces for all ages.

IV. Benefits of cognitive stimulation applications

1. Accessibility and flexibility

- **Home use**: Training at any time, anywhere.
- **Adapted to individual pace**: freedom to choose the length and frequency of sessions.

2. Greater commitment

- **Fun aspect**: Games and challenges make training more enjoyable.
- **Motivation**: Visible progress encourages perseverance.

3. Customize your exercises

- **Tailor-made programs**: adapted to the user's specific needs and objectives.
- **Continuous evolution**: Automatic difficulty level adjustment to maintain the challenge.

4. Follow-up by healthcare professionals

- **Data sharing** : Results can be communicated to therapists or physicians.
- **Complementing traditional therapies**: Integration into cognitive rehabilitation programs.

V. Limitations and considerations

1. Variable efficiency

- **Lack of solid scientific evidence**: Some applications have not been the subject of rigorous studies demonstrating their effectiveness.

- **Generalization of benefits**: Improvements may not translate into gains in everyday life.

2. **Dependence on technology**

    - **Limited access**: Compatible device and Internet connection required.
    - **Digital skills**: Elderly people may find it difficult to use computers.

3. **Cost**

    - **Paid subscriptions** : Some applications require a purchase or subscription to access full functionality.
    - **Advertising and integrated purchases**: Possible presence of advertising or incentives for additional purchases.

4. **Data protection**

    - **Confidentiality**: Risks associated with the collection and storage of personal information.
    - **Regulatory compliance**: Importance of checking that the application complies with data protection standards, such as the RGPD.

VI. Tips for choosing a cognitive stimulation application

1. **Define your goals**

    - **Identify areas for improvement**: memory, attention, language, etc.
    - **Set realistic expectations**: Understand that applications are just one tool among many.

2. **Checking reliability**

    - **Look for scientifically validated applications**: Prefer those supported by studies or developed with experts.
    - **Consult reviews**: Read feedback from other users and professional recommendations.

3. **Test several options**

    - **Try out the free versions**: Before making a financial commitment, test the interface and exercises offered.
    - **Evaluate usability**: Make sure the application is pleasant and easy to use.

4. **Consult a healthcare professional**

    - **Ask for advice**: Doctors, neuropsychologists and speech therapists can recommend suitable applications.
    - **Integrate the application into an overall program**: use it as a complement to other activities or therapies.

VII. Future prospects

1. **Artificial intelligence and greater personalization**

    - **Real-time adaptation**: using AI to adjust exercises according to instantaneous performance.
    - **Predictive analysis**: Anticipating future needs and preventing cognitive decline.

2. **Virtual and augmented reality**

    - **Total immersion**: Creating stimulating environments for a more engaging experience.

    - **Therapeutic applications**: Use for rehabilitation after stroke or head injury.
3. **Integration with other devices**
    - **Biometric sensors**: heart rate and sleep monitoring for a holistic approach.
    - **Brain-computer interfaces**: Perspectives for people with severe disabilities.

Assistance robots

- Companion robots to combat isolation

Social isolation is a growing problem in modern society, particularly affecting the elderly, people with disabilities and those living alone. This isolation can have harmful consequences on mental and physical health, increasing the risk of depression, anxiety and chronic illness. Faced with this challenge, companion robots are emerging as an innovative solution to provide support, companionship and improve quality of life for isolated people. This article explores the role of companion robots in combating isolation, their functionalities, benefits, associated challenges and future prospects.

I. What is a companion robot?

1. **Definition**
    A companion robot is a robotic device designed to interact socially with humans, by mimicking certain aspects of human or animal behavior. These robots are programmed to communicate, respond to stimuli and, in some cases, learn from interactions with their users.

2. Types of companion robots

- **Anthropomorphic robots**: Resemble humans, with facial expressions and articulated movements.
- **Zoomorphic robots**: Imitate animals such as dogs, cats and seals.
- **Non-morphic robots**: have an abstract appearance but are capable of rich social interaction.

II. Companion robot features

1. Social interaction

    - **Verbal communication**: Ability to speak, understand and respond to users.
    - **Emotional expressions**: Display emotions through facial expressions, sounds or movements.
    - **Face and voice recognition**: Identify users to personalize interactions.

2. Daily assistance

    - **Reminders**: Notifications for medication, appointments or activities.
    - **Mobility assistance**: Assistance with moving around or carrying small objects.
    - **Information**: Provision of news, weather and other useful information.

3. Entertainment and cognitive stimulation

    - **Interactive games**: To stimulate memory and thinking, or simply to entertain.
    - **Reading**: Recitation of books, poems or music.

- **Physical activities**: Encouragement to exercise or dance.

4. **Health monitoring**

    - **Vital signs monitoring**: Measurement of heart rate, blood pressure, etc.
    - **Fall detection**: Accident alert for rapid intervention.
    - **Communication with caregivers**: Passing on information to relatives or healthcare professionals.

III. Benefits of companion robots in the fight against isolation

1. **Reduces feelings of loneliness**

    - **Constant presence**: Robots offer uninterrupted companionship, reducing the feeling of being alone.
    - **Regular interaction**: shared conversations and activities strengthen the social bond.

2. **Improving mental health**

    - **Emotional support**: robots can detect emotions and provide comfort.
    - **Cognitive stimulation**: Games and discussions help keep cognitive functions active.

3. **Increased autonomy**

    - **Help with daily tasks**: Facilitates daily life without constant dependence on a third party.
    - **Encouraging activity**: Encouraging participation in physical or social activities.

4. **Support for caregivers**

    - **Lightening the load**: Robots can take over certain routine tasks, allowing caregivers to concentrate on other aspects.
    - **Remote monitoring**: Provide updates on user status to families or professionals.

IV. Examples of companion robots

1. **Paro**

    - **Description**: Interactive seal-shaped robot designed for animal-assisted therapy.
    - **Features**: Reacts to touch, light, sound, temperature and posture. It emits sounds and movements to interact with the user.
    - **Use**: Effective in reducing stress and anxiety in elderly people with dementia.

2. **Pepper**

    - **Description**: A humanoid robot capable of recognizing human emotions.
    - **Features**: Communicates verbally, recognizes faces, can initiate conversations and provide information.
    - **Use**: Used in hospitals, retirement homes and shopping malls to interact with people.

3. **Buddy**

    - **Description**: Social robot developed to assist families and individuals.
    - **Features**: Interacts with family members, controls home automation devices, monitors the home and provides emotional support.

- **Use**: Aims to be a family companion for all generations.

V. Challenges and considerations

1. **Ethical aspects**

    - **Emotional attachment**: Risk of users developing excessive attachment, which can affect real human relationships.
    - **Replacing human interaction**: Robots must not completely replace human contact, which is essential for well-being.

2. **Data confidentiality and security**

    - **Collection of personal information**: Need to protect sensitive data collected by robots.
    - **Cyber-security**: Risks of hacking that could compromise the user's privacy or security.

3. **Social acceptance**

    - **Resistance to change**: Some users may be reluctant to interact with robots.
    - **Stigmatization**: the risk of robots being perceived negatively, as a sign of weakness or abandonment.

4. **Cost and accessibility**

    - **High price**: Companion robots can be expensive, limiting their accessibility.
    - **Maintenance and support**: You need reliable maintenance services to keep things running smoothly.

VI. Future prospects

1. **Technological advances**

    - **Improved artificial intelligence**: better understanding of natural language, emotions and human behavior.
    - **Machine learning**: the ability of robots to learn and adapt to individual preferences.

2. **Integration into healthcare systems**

    - **Pilot programs** : Expansion of projects involving robots in retirement homes and hospitals.
    - **Collaboration with caregivers**: Robots as complementary tools for healthcare professionals.

3. **Cost reduction**

    - **Mass production**: Increased production can lead to lower prices.
    - **Public and private funding**: Investments to make these technologies more accessible.

4. **Cultural acceptance**

    - **Awareness**: Education on the benefits and limitations of companion robots.
    - **Cultural customization**: adapting robots to different cultures and languages for greater acceptance.

- Future prospects for robotics in geriatrics

The aging of the population is a global phenomenon that poses major challenges for healthcare systems. In geriatrics, the growing demand for personalized care and support for the elderly calls for innovative solutions. Robotics is emerging as a promising answer to improving the quality of life, autonomy and well-being of the elderly. Technological advances in artificial intelligence, mechatronics and communication are paving the way for a new generation of robots adapted to the specific needs of the elderly. This talk explores the future prospects of robotics in geriatrics, focusing on potential innovations, challenges and the impact on patients and healthcare professionals.

I. The current state of robotics in geriatrics

1. Physical assistance robots

- **Exoskeletons**: Wearable devices that increase muscle strength, helping the elderly to walk or stand.
- **Handling robots**: Help caregivers move patients safely, reducing the risk of injury.

2. Companion robots

- **Social robots**: like Paro the seal or Pepper, which interact with patients to reduce isolation and stimulate social interaction.
- **Cognitive stimulation**: Robots offering games and activities to maintain cognitive function.

3. Telehealth robots

- **Telepresence**: enabling doctors and families to communicate with patients at a distance.
- **Home monitoring**: Sensors and robots that monitor vital signs and daily activities.

II. Technological innovations and future trends

1. Advanced AI integration

- **Machine learning**: robots will be able to adapt to patients' habits and preferences.
- **Natural language processing**: Improving human-robot communication for more natural interactions.

2. Versatile humanoid robots

- **Assistance with daily activities**: Help with meal preparation, personal hygiene and household chores.
- **Enriched social interaction**: Ability to recognize emotions and respond empathetically.

3. Rehabilitation robotics

- **Assisted physical therapy**: Robots that guide movements for motor rehabilitation.
- **Cognitive re-education**: interactive programs to improve memory and attention.

4. Robotic systems integrated into infrastructures

- **Smart homes**: Integrating robots with home automation systems for a safe, adapted environment.
- **Autonomous transport:** robotized vehicles to make it easier for the elderly to get around.

5. Medical nanorobotics

- **Precise diagnostics**: Nanorobots capable of detecting anomalies at the cellular level.
- **Targeted therapies**: Precise administration of drugs to treat specific conditions.

III - Impact on quality of care and autonomy

1. Patient empowerment

- **Increased independence**: Robots enable the elderly to perform tasks without constant human assistance.
- **Personalized care**: Tailoring services to individual needs.

2. Improving the quality of care

- **Continuous monitoring**: Early detection of health problems thanks to 24-hour monitoring.
- **Reducing errors**: Robotic assistance in medication and treatment management.

3. Support for caregivers

- **Reduced workload**: Robots take on repetitive or physically demanding tasks.
- **Prevention of musculoskeletal disorders**: Reducing physical effort for caregivers.

4. Social and cognitive stimulation

- **Emotional commitment**: Companion robots encourage interaction and reduce feelings of loneliness.
- **Enriching activities**: Educational and entertaining programs to maintain mental acuity.

IV. Challenges and ethical considerations

1. Acceptance by patients and staff

- **User receptiveness**: Need to ensure that patients are comfortable with the robots.

- **Staff training**: Preparing caregivers to work with robotic technologies.

2. **Ethical and social issues**

    - **Dehumanization of care**: the risk of technology replacing essential human contact.
    - **Confidentiality and data protection**: Security of information collected by robots.

3. **Financial accessibility**

    - **High cost of technology**: risk of unequal access for less affluent patients.
    - **Financing models** : Solutions needed to make robotics accessible to all.

4. **Regulatory and legal framework**

    - **Safety standards**: Setting standards to ensure robot reliability.
    - **Liability**: Clarification of responsibilities in the event of malfunction or accident.

V. Research and development prospects

1. **Technological innovation**

    - **Improving robots' cognitive capabilities**: Developing more advanced artificial intelligence.
    - **Miniaturization and mobility**: creating smaller, more mobile robots for better integration.

2. **Interdisciplinary collaboration**

    - **Engineering and healthcare**: cooperation between technicians, doctors and carers to design adapted robots.

- **Patient involvement**: Involve end-users in the development process.

3. **Clinical studies and validation**
   - **Evidence-based research**: Evaluating the effectiveness of robots in real-life contexts.
   - **Feedback**: Using feedback from patients and caregivers to fine-tune technologies.

4. **Education and awareness**
   - **Training programs**: Preparing healthcare professionals to use robotics.
   - **Raising public awareness**: Information on the benefits and limitations of robots in geriatrics.

VI. Impact on the healthcare system

1. **Reorganization of care services**
   - **Integrating robots into protocols**: Adapting clinical practices to include robotics.
   - **New professional roles**: the emergence of medical robotics specialists.

2. **Economic efficiency**
   - **Long-term cost reduction**: fewer hospital admissions and optimized use of resources.
   - **Workforce management**: automating the response to nursing shortages.

3. **Improving home care**
   - **Deinstitutionalization**: Enabling the elderly to remain in their own homes for longer.
   - **Support for family caregivers**: Provide tools to facilitate home care.

Chapter 8

Patient Autonomy and Health Promotion

Prevention of Age-Related Pathologies

- Recommended vaccinations

Vaccination is one of the most significant advances in modern medicine, having saved millions of lives by preventing serious infectious diseases. It is an essential public health tool, not only to protect individuals, but also to ensure the health security of the community. Vaccine recommendations evolve in line with scientific advances, disease epidemiology and health policies. So it's important to keep up to date with recommended vaccines at every stage of life.

The importance of vaccination

Vaccines stimulate the immune system to recognize and fight specific infectious agents. By developing immunity without having to experience the disease, individuals are protected against potentially fatal or disabling infections. In addition, high vaccination coverage in the population contributes to herd immunity, reducing the circulation of pathogens and protecting the most vulnerable people who cannot be vaccinated for medical reasons.

Recommended vaccinations for infants and children

From birth, infants are exposed to a variety of pathogens. The vaccination schedule is designed to offer early protection against the most dangerous diseases.

- **Hepatitis B**: Administered from birth, this vaccine protects against the hepatitis B virus, responsible for chronic liver infections that can lead to cirrhosis or liver cancer.

- **Diphtheria, Tetanus, Pertussis (DTPaP)**: This combined vaccine is given at 2, 4 and 11 months, with booster doses at age 6. Diphtheria and tetanus are serious diseases caused by bacterial toxins, while pertussis is a highly contagious respiratory infection.

- **Haemophilus influenzae type b (Hib)**: Administered at the same time as DTPaP, it protects against invasive infections such as meningitis and epiglottitis.

- **Pneumococcus**: This vaccine protects against Streptococcus pneumoniae, responsible for pneumonia, meningitis and otitis. It is administered at 2, 4 and 11 months.

- **Poliomyelitis (IPV)**: Polio is a viral disease that can lead to irreversible paralysis. The inactivated vaccine is administered at the same time as DTPaP.

- **Measles, Mumps, Rubella (MMR)**: This trivalent vaccine is given at 12 months, with a second dose between 16 and 18 months. These viral diseases can lead to serious complications, particularly neurological.

- **Meningococcal C**: Vaccination against meningococcal C, which causes meningitis and fulminant septicemia, is recommended at 5 months, with a booster at 12 months.

Vaccinations recommended for adolescents

Adolescence is a key period for booster vaccinations and the introduction of new protection products.

- **Diphtheria, Tetanus, Pertussis, Poliomyelitis (dTcaP) booster**: A booster is recommended at age 11-13 to maintain optimal protection.

- **Human Papillomavirus (HPV)**: Recommended for girls and boys between the ages of 11 and 14, with catch-up vaccination possible up to age 19, this vaccine protects against HPV infections responsible for cervical, anal and other genital cancers.

- **Meningococcal ACWY**: A quadrivalent vaccine is recommended in adolescence to extend protection against other strains of meningococcus.

Recommended vaccinations for adults

Adults must also keep their vaccinations up to date to protect themselves and prevent the transmission of disease.

- **DTP boosters**: Boosters are recommended at ages 25, 45 and 65, then every 10 years for tetanus, diphtheria and polio.

- **Whooping cough**: A booster in adulthood, especially for future parents and healthcare professionals, helps protect infants who have not yet been vaccinated.

- **Seasonal influenza**: Recommended every year for people over 65, pregnant women, people with certain chronic diseases and healthcare professionals.

- **Shingles**: A vaccine is available for people aged 65 to 74 to prevent shingles and its painful complications.

- **COVID-19**: Recommendations evolve according to the epidemic situation, but vaccination remains strongly encouraged for all adults, with booster doses according to official guidelines.

Vaccinations for at-risk populations

Some people are at increased risk of infection and require specific vaccinations.

- **Immunocompromised people**: Appropriate vaccinations are recommended according to their state of health and treatment.

- **Pregnant women**: Vaccination against influenza and whooping cough is recommended to protect both mother and newborn.

- **Healthcare professionals**: Must be up to date with vaccinations to avoid nosocomial transmission.

- **Travelers**: Depending on the destination, specific vaccines such as yellow fever, typhoid or Japanese encephalitis may be required.

The importance of vaccination coverage

High vaccination coverage is essential to prevent epidemics. Herd immunity protects unvaccinated individuals, such as newborn babies or immunocompromised people. Vaccination campaigns have eradicated smallpox and are close to eliminating polio. However, the resurgence of certain diseases, such as measles, reminds us of the need to maintain vigilance and sufficient vaccination coverage.

Preconceived ideas and vaccine hesitancy

Despite scientific proof of the efficacy and safety of vaccines, misconceptions persist, fuelling vaccine hesitancy. It's important to seek information from reliable sources, and to consult healthcare professionals for accurate answers to questions and concerns.

- Early detection of chronic diseases

Early detection of chronic diseases is a major public health issue, aimed at identifying conditions at an early stage, before the onset of significant symptoms. This proactive approach not only improves the prognosis of patients, but also reduces the costs associated with long-term treatment and eases the burden on the healthcare system. Chronic diseases such as diabetes, hypertension, cardiovascular disease and certain cancers can benefit greatly from early detection, paving the way for early and effective interventions.

Early detection relies on the use of specific screening tests, adapted to each disease and target population. These tests are generally simple, minimally invasive and accessible, making them widely available to the public. For example, regular measurement of blood pressure can reveal hypertension before it causes damage to vital organs. Similarly, blood tests can detect elevated glucose levels, indicating potential diabetes.

The importance of early detection lies in its ability to prevent the serious complications associated with chronic diseases. By identifying a condition at an asymptomatic stage, healthcare professionals can introduce therapeutic or preventive measures that slow or halt disease progression. In the case of colorectal cancer, for example, colonoscopy screening can detect precancerous polyps, enabling them to be removed before they develop into malignant tumors.

Early detection also helps to improve patients' quality of life. By avoiding the onset of disabling symptoms or irreversible complications, individuals can maintain an active and productive life. This has a positive impact not only personally, but also socio-economically, by reducing absenteeism from work and dependence on long-term care.

To be effective, screening must be targeted and organized. Mass screening programs are set up for certain diseases, based on epidemiological and economic criteria. For example, organized mammography screening for breast cancer is offered to women aged between 50 and 74, the age at highest risk. Similarly, cervical smear screening is recommended for women aged 25 and over.

Public awareness is an essential component of successful early detection. Informing the population about the risks, predisposing factors and benefits of screening encourages individuals to actively participate in their own health. Information campaigns, prevention initiatives and the involvement of primary care professionals, such as general practitioners, play a crucial role in this process.

It's also important to consider the potential barriers to screening. Fear of diagnosis, lack of information, geographical or financial constraints may dissuade some people from undergoing screening. Health policies must therefore incorporate measures to make screening accessible to all, notably by offering free tests or organizing mobile campaigns in rural areas.

Personalized screening is an emerging trend, made possible by technological advances and a growing understanding of genetics. Genetic testing can identify individuals at high risk of developing certain diseases, such as breast cancer linked to BRCA1 and BRCA2 mutations. This approach enables screening and preventive measures to be tailored to each individual's profile, improving the effectiveness of interventions.

However, early detection is not without its challenges. There is a risk of false positives, leading to unnecessary further investigations and patient anxiety. Conversely, false negatives can give false confidence and delay diagnosis. It is therefore essential that screening tests are scientifically validated for their reliability, and that healthcare professionals are trained to interpret results appropriately.

The ethics of screening must also be taken into account. Respect for informed consent, confidentiality of results and the right not to know are fundamental principles. Patients must be informed of the implications of testing, the possible consequences of early diagnosis and the options available to them.

- Promoting a healthy lifestyle

Promoting a healthy lifestyle is essential for improving individual health and well-being, as well as preventing many chronic diseases. Adopting healthy habits has a positive influence on all aspects of life, including physical, mental and social health. It is therefore crucial to understand the components of a healthy lifestyle and how to promote it effectively within the population.

A healthy lifestyle rests on several fundamental pillars. Firstly, a balanced diet is essential to provide the body with the nutrients it needs to function properly. Eating a variety of foods rich in vitamins, minerals, fiber and other nutrients promotes cardiovascular health, boosts the immune system and helps maintain a healthy body weight. Fruits and vegetables, whole grains, lean proteins and healthy fats are recommended, while limiting the intake of added sugars, salt and saturated fats.

Regular physical activity is another key element of a healthy lifestyle. Exercise helps to strengthen the cardiovascular system, improve muscle strength, flexibility and endurance, and reduce the risk of diseases such as diabetes, obesity and certain cancers. Physical activity also has beneficial effects on mental health, reducing stress, anxiety and depression. Adults are advised to engage in at least 150 minutes of moderate-intensity activity per week, such as brisk walking, cycling or swimming.

Sleep also plays a crucial role in maintaining good health. Adequate rest allows the body to regenerate, supports immune system function and promotes mental health. Adults should aim for between seven and nine hours' sleep a night. To improve sleep quality, it's important to establish a regular routine, create an environment conducive to rest and avoid stimulants such as caffeine or screens before bedtime.

Stress management is an essential component of a healthy lifestyle. Chronic stress can have detrimental effects on physical and mental health, increasing the risk of cardiovascular disease, sleep disorders and mental health problems. Techniques such as meditation, deep breathing, yoga or the practice of relaxing activities can help reduce stress and improve overall well-being.

Avoiding risky behavior is also fundamental to preserving health. This includes limiting or abstaining from the consumption of tobacco, alcohol and psychoactive substances. Smoking is one of the main causes of preventable diseases such as cancer, lung and cardiovascular disease. Similarly, excessive alcohol consumption can damage the liver, increase the risk of cancer and contribute to social and psychological problems.

Positive social relationships and community support play an important role in promoting a healthy lifestyle. Participating in social activities, maintaining friendships and strong family relationships contribute to emotional well-being and can even have beneficial effects on physical health. Community involvement, volunteering and group activities can reinforce a sense of belonging and personal satisfaction.

To effectively promote a healthy lifestyle, it's important to adopt a comprehensive approach that includes education, accessibility and support. Awareness campaigns can inform the public about the benefits of healthy habits and how to integrate them into daily life. Educational programs in schools, workplaces and communities can teach the skills needed to make informed health choices.

Accessibility of resources is also crucial. This means ensuring that individuals have access to affordable, healthy food, safe spaces for physical activity, and quality health services. Public policy can play a role by supporting initiatives such as the creation of bicycle paths, the development of parks, the regulation of advertising for unhealthy foods and the introduction of smoking cessation support programs.

Social and environmental support is essential to encourage behavior change. Individuals are more likely to adopt and maintain healthy habits when they are supported by those around them, and when their environment facilitates these choices. Support groups, community programs and family initiatives can help create a culture of positive health.

Social and therapeutic leisure activities

- The importance of recreational activities for well-being

Recreational activities occupy an essential place in daily life, providing a balance between professional, family and personal obligations. They are much more than mere pastimes; they are a fundamental pillar of physical, mental and emotional well-being. By engaging in leisure activities that provide pleasure and satisfaction, individuals strengthen their overall health and improve their quality of life.

On the physical front, recreational activities such as sports, dancing and hiking help to maintain good physical condition. They help strengthen muscles, improve blood circulation and increase endurance. Physical exercise releases endorphins, often referred to as "happy hormones", which induce a feeling of well-being and reduce stress. By making these activities a regular part of their routine, people can prevent various diseases linked to a sedentary lifestyle, such as cardiovascular disorders and diabetes.

Beyond the physical benefits, recreational activities play a crucial role in mental health. They offer an escape from everyday stresses, helping to relieve accumulated pressure. Taking up a creative hobby, such as painting, music or writing, stimulates the imagination and encourages self-expression. These activities encourage concentration and mindfulness, helping to reduce anxiety and negative thoughts. What's more, they can boost self-esteem and confidence in one's abilities, providing a sense of personal accomplishment.

Social interaction is also at the heart of recreational activities. Participating in sports clubs, reading groups or art workshops creates opportunities to meet new people and forge bonds. These social relationships enrich life, provide support and reinforce the sense of belonging to a community. They are particularly important in the fight against isolation and loneliness, factors that can adversely affect mental and emotional health.

Leisure activities also foster the development of skills and knowledge. Learning a new language, taking up photography or cooking classes broadens horizons and nourishes intellectual curiosity. This ongoing learning stimulates the brain, helping to maintain cognitive function and prevent age-related decline. They also encourage adaptability and resilience, valuable qualities in a constantly changing world.

Recreational activities can also serve as a means of discovering and appreciating nature. Outdoor activities such as gardening, camping or birdwatching strengthen the bond with the environment and raise awareness of its protection. Contact with nature has soothing effects, reducing stress and improving mood. It also promotes greater self-awareness and a broader perspective on life.

It's important to recognize that recreational activities are not a luxury, but a necessity for a healthy life balance. They recharge batteries, increase personal satisfaction and boost motivation in other areas of life. Employers and educational institutions can contribute to this approach by encouraging a balance between work and personal life, offering dedicated spaces for recreation or organizing social events.

To maximize the benefits of recreational activities, it's essential to choose hobbies that match your interests and passions.

Everyone is unique, and what gives pleasure to one person may not suit another. So it's a good idea to explore different activities to find those that resonate most with your personal preferences. These can include individual or team sports, creative arts, board games, travel or any other activity that brings joy.

- Organization of workshops and outings

The organization of workshops and outings is an essential component in enriching the personal and social experience of individuals, be they children, teenagers, adults or the elderly. These activities foster learning, stimulate creativity, strengthen social ties and promote general well-being. By setting up interactive workshops and educational or recreational outings, we create unique opportunities to explore new horizons, acquire skills and forge meaningful relationships.

Workshop planning starts with identifying the needs and interests of the target audience. Understanding participants' aspirations is crucial to proposing activities that engage and motivate them. For example, for children, artistic workshops such as painting, modeling or music can awaken their creativity and develop their talents. For adults, personal development, cooking or DIY workshops offer opportunities to learn new skills while socializing.

Once the themes have been chosen, it's important to select skilled and passionate facilitators. These professionals or volunteers play a key role in the success of the workshop, creating a welcoming environment and adapting their approach to the needs of the participants. They must be able to pass on their knowledge in an accessible and interactive way, encouraging everyone's active participation.

The logistical aspect is also fundamental. You need to choose a suitable, comfortable venue equipped with the necessary materials. Safety must be a priority, especially if the workshop involves manual or physical activities. It's also important to set times that suit the participants, taking into account their personal or professional constraints.

Communication around the workshop is essential to ensure good participation. Using different channels, such as social networks, posters, newsletters or word-of-mouth, you can reach a wide audience. It's a good idea to provide clear information about the workshop's content, objectives, registration procedures and any participation fees.

When it comes to organizing outings, these offer an opportunity to discover new environments, open up to different cultures and broaden horizons. Whether it's a visit to a museum, a nature hike, a show or a cultural trip, outings enrich participants' experience and create lasting memories.

Preparing an outing requires careful attention to detail. First, you need to define the purpose of the outing: is it educational, recreational, sporting or cultural? Next, the destination or activity must be chosen according to the group's interests and abilities. For example, for a group of elderly people, a guided tour of a historic site with easy access will be more appropriate than a mountain hike.

Logistical aspects include booking transport, purchasing tickets, planning meals and arranging accommodation if necessary. Safety is paramount: you need to arrange insurance, inform participants of safety instructions and ensure that the sites visited comply with current standards.

Communication prior to the outing is crucial to inform participants of the practical details: times, meeting points, equipment to bring, weather conditions, etc. Providing a detailed program helps participants to prepare and enjoy the experience to the full.

During the outing, competent supervisors ensure that the activity runs smoothly. They're there to answer questions, deal with the unexpected and ensure group cohesion. A caring and dynamic attitude on their part helps to create a convivial atmosphere and encourage exchanges between participants.

After the workshop or outing, it's a good idea to gather feedback from participants. Feedback helps to assess satisfaction, identify strengths and areas for improvement. This helps to adapt future activities so that they meet the public's expectations even better.

- Collaboration with animators and volunteers

Collaboration with animators and volunteers is essential to the success of many community projects and initiatives. Whether it's organizing cultural events, educational workshops, sports activities or social initiatives, the synergy between the various players helps maximize the impact of the efforts deployed. This cooperation not only promotes operational efficiency, but also strengthens the social fabric by creating solid bonds between community members.

Leaders play a key role in the implementation of activities. They are often the driving force that breathes energy and dynamism into projects. Thanks to their pedagogical skills, creativity and ability to motivate participants, they make the activities attractive and rewarding. Volunteers, for their part, contribute their time, enthusiasm and varied skills. Their selfless commitment is an invaluable asset in extending the reach of our initiatives to a wider audience.

Collaboration between organizers, animators and volunteers is based on open and transparent communication. It's important to clearly define project objectives, roles and responsibilities. An initial meeting helps to share the overall vision, listen to ideas and suggestions, and align expectations. This collective planning phase promotes ownership of the project by all team members and stimulates motivation.

Drawing up a detailed action plan makes it easier to coordinate efforts. By defining specific tasks, deadlines and resource requirements, misunderstandings and duplication of effort are avoided. Project management tools, such as shared calendars or online collaboration platforms, can be used to ensure effective follow-up and fluid communication. It is also beneficial to schedule regular checkpoints to assess project progress and make any necessary adjustments.

Training and support for facilitators and volunteers are crucial to the success of the collaboration. Offering training sessions helps to develop the necessary skills and ensure that everyone involved is well prepared for their respective missions. This can include training in facilitation techniques, group management, first aid or the handling of specific equipment. By providing the right tools and knowledge, the confidence of volunteers and leaders is strengthened, resulting in better quality activities.

Recognition of the work accomplished by animators and volunteers is essential to maintain their commitment and motivation. Simple gestures, such as expressing gratitude at meetings, offering certificates of recognition or organizing thank-you events, can have a significant impact on team morale. Valuing their contribution shows that their work is appreciated and encourages future participation.

Working with animators and volunteers is not without its challenges. Differences of opinion, scheduling conflicts or differences in working styles can arise. To overcome these obstacles, it's important to adopt an empathetic approach and foster a climate of mutual respect. Establishing effective communication channels helps to resolve problems quickly and maintain a positive team dynamic.

Involving volunteers and animators in the decision-making process can also strengthen collaboration. Inviting them to share their ideas and perspectives enriches the project and encourages a sense of co-responsibility. This participatory approach fosters innovation and can lead to creative solutions for achieving the set objectives.

Collaboration with animators and volunteers has positive spin-offs that go beyond the project itself. It contributes to strengthening social cohesion, developing human capital and building more resilient communities. Participants in activities benefit from the expertise and commitment of facilitators and volunteers, enriching their experience and fostering their personal development.

Chapter 9

Management of Cognitive and Behavioral Disorders

A closer look at dementia

- Differentiating between types of dementia

Dementia is a general term that describes a progressive deterioration in cognitive functions, affecting memory, reasoning, behavior and the ability to carry out daily activities. However, there are several types of dementia, each with distinct causes, symptoms and course. Understanding these differences is essential for accurate diagnosis and appropriate care.

Alzheimer's disease

Alzheimer's disease is the most common form of dementia, accounting for around 60-70% of cases. It is characterized by a progressive loss of memory, often starting with difficulty remembering recent events. Symptoms also include language disorders, disorientation in time and space, judgment problems and personality changes.

Biologically, the disease is associated with the accumulation of beta-amyloid plaques and neurofibrillary tangles of tau protein in the brain, leading to neuronal death. Evolution is generally slow but progressive, leading to total dependence in advanced stages.

Vascular dementia

Vascular dementia is the second most common form. It results from damage to the brain caused by disturbances in blood circulation, such as strokes or micro-infarcts. Symptoms vary according to the areas of the brain affected, but often include impaired attention, planning and memory.

Unlike Alzheimer's disease, vascular dementia can have a sudden onset and a stepwise progression, linked to new vascular events. Risk factors include high blood pressure, diabetes, smoking and hypercholesterolemia.

Lewy body dementia

Lewy body dementia is characterized by the presence of abnormal deposits of proteins called Lewy bodies in brain cells. Symptoms include pronounced cognitive fluctuations, detailed and recurrent visual hallucinations, and motor symptoms similar to those of Parkinson's disease, such as rigidity and tremors.

Patients may also experience sleep disturbances, increased sensitivity to neuroleptics and fainting. Progression is generally rapid, and diagnosis can be difficult due to similarities with other neurodegenerative diseases.

Frontotemporal dementia

Frontotemporal dementia mainly affects the frontal and temporal lobes of the brain, responsible for behavior, personality and language. It often occurs in younger people, between the ages of 45 and 65.

Symptoms include marked personality changes, such as disinhibition, apathy, inappropriate social behaviour and language disorders (aphasia). Short-term memory is generally preserved in the early stages. The course varies, but the disease inevitably progresses to severe deterioration of cognitive functions.

Parkinson's disease with dementia

In some patients with Parkinson's disease, dementia can develop, usually in the advanced stages. Symptoms include impaired memory, attention, judgment and word-finding. The motor symptoms of Parkinson's disease, such as tremors, rigidity and slowness of movement, are also present.

Differentiation from Lewy body dementia can be tricky, but is often based on the time lag between onset of cognitive symptoms and motor symptoms.

Creutzfeldt-Jakob disease

Creutzfeldt-Jakob disease is a rare, rapidly progressive form of dementia caused by prions, abnormal infectious proteins. Symptoms include rapidly progressive dementia, motor disorders, myoclonus (involuntary muscle twitching) and visual changes. The disease is fatal, usually within a year of the onset of symptoms.

Hydrocephalus at normal pressure

This condition is caused by an accumulation of cerebrospinal fluid in the cerebral ventricles, resulting in pressure on brain tissue. The main symptoms are unsteady gait, urinary incontinence and cognitive impairment. Early diagnosis is crucial, as surgical treatment (placement of a shunt) can improve symptoms.

Mixed dementia

Mixed dementia refers to the simultaneous presence of several types of dementia, often Alzheimer's disease combined with vascular dementia. Symptoms reflect a combination of disorders present in each type, which can complicate diagnosis and management.

Clinical differentiation and diagnosis

To differentiate between the different types of dementia, a full assessment is required:

- **Detailed history**: Including medical and family history, and chronology of symptoms.
- **Neurological examination**: Assessment of cognitive, motor and sensory functions.
- **Neuropsychological tests**: To identify specific cognitive profiles.

- **Brain imaging**: MRI or CT scan to detect structural abnormalities.
- **Biological tests**: To rule out reversible causes (vitamin deficiencies, thyroid disorders).
- **Lumbar puncture**: In some cases, to analyze cerebrospinal fluid.

The importance of differentiation

Distinguishing between the different types of dementia is essential for :

- **Adapting treatment**: Some drugs are specific to certain forms of dementia.
- **Prognosis**: Progression and life expectancy vary according to type.
- **Care planning**: Anticipating support and assistance needs.
- **Advising families**: Particularly for hereditary forms, such as certain frontotemporal dementias.

- Symptoms and disease stages

Alzheimer's disease and other forms of dementia are progressive neurodegenerative disorders that lead to a gradual deterioration in cognitive, behavioral and physical functions. Understanding the progression of symptoms and the stages of the disease is essential for appropriate management, enabling patients and their families to prepare for the challenges ahead and put in place effective support strategies.

Early stage (light stage)

In the early stages of the disease, symptoms are often subtle and may be mistaken for the normal effects of aging or stress. People may have difficulty remembering recent events or newly learned information. For example, they may forget recent conversations, misplace common objects such as keys, or have difficulty remembering appointments.

Attention and concentration problems become more apparent. The person may have difficulty following the thread of a conversation or reading. Difficulties in performing familiar tasks begin to appear, especially those requiring planning or organization, such as preparing a complex meal or managing finances.

Emotionally, changes may occur, such as increased irritability, anxiety or mild depression. Awareness of one's own difficulties can lead to frustration and embarrassment, causing some individuals to withdraw socially to avoid embarrassment.

Intermediate stage (moderate stage)

As the disease progresses, symptoms become more pronounced and begin to interfere significantly with daily life. Memory problems worsen, affecting not only recent memories, but also past events. The person may forget important personal information, such as their address or the names of close relatives.

Language skills are affected. Difficulties in finding the right words, following conversations or understanding complex instructions become apparent. This can lead to frustrating communication for the patient and those around him/her.

Disorientation in time and space becomes more frequent. The person may get lost in familiar places, fail to recognize familiar locations, or forget the date and season. Impaired judgment and decision-making intensify, which can lead to inappropriate or dangerous behavior, such as crossing the street without looking or handling money irresponsibly.

Changes in behavior and personality are common at this stage. The individual may exhibit agitation, aggression, distrust or hallucinations. They may also develop repetitive or compulsive habits, such as constantly putting things away.

Daily activities are becoming increasingly difficult. Dressing, bathing, preparing meals or managing household chores often require assistance. Dependence on caregivers increases, and the need for constant supervision becomes apparent to ensure the patient's safety.

Advanced stage (severe stage)

In the final stage of the disease, cognitive and physical deterioration is profound. The person loses the ability to communicate coherently, with speech limited to simple words or phrases, or becomes non-verbal. Language comprehension is also severely impaired.

Memory is severely affected. Patients no longer recognize family members, close friends or even their own reflection in the mirror. Personal memories and knowledge acquired throughout life are almost completely lost.

Motor skills decline. The person may have difficulty walking, sitting or maintaining balance. In later stages, they often become bedridden or wheelchair-bound. Coordination and fine motor skills are compromised, making it impossible to perform simple gestures such as holding a spoon.

Bodily functions are disrupted. The person may lose sphincter control, requiring assistance with personal hygiene. Swallowing problems appear, increasing the risk of malnutrition and pulmonary aspiration.

The immune system is weakened, making the patient more vulnerable to infections such as pneumonia or urinary tract infections. The general fragility of the body leads to a deterioration in overall health.

General considerations on disease progression

It's important to note that the course of the disease and the progression of symptoms can vary considerably from person to person. Some patients may go through the stages more quickly, while others may maintain stable functioning for several years. Factors such as age, general state of health, level of intellectual and social activity, as well as therapeutic interventions, can influence the course of the disease.

Impact on family members and caregivers

The progression of the disease has a significant impact on family members and caregivers. The increasing demands of caregiving can lead to physical and emotional stress, fatigue and an increased risk of depression. Support for caregivers, whether through community resources, support groups or respite services, is essential to maintaining their own health and well-being.

Management strategies

In the early stages, non-pharmacological interventions can be implemented to support the patient's remaining abilities. These include cognitive stimulation activities, the establishment of structured routines and the use of mnemonic aids, such as diaries or visual reminders.

Drug treatments can help alleviate certain cognitive or behavioral symptoms, although they cannot halt the progression of the disease. Multidisciplinary management, involving doctors, nurses, occupational therapists and other healthcare professionals, is recommended to meet the patient's complex needs.

Adapting the environment is also crucial to ensuring the patient's safety and comfort. This can include removing obstacles to mobility, installing safety devices and simplifying the living space.

Preparing for the future

From the earliest stages, it's important to discuss future plans with the patient and family. This may include decisions on end-of-life care, advance directives, legal and financial aspects. Addressing these issues early helps to respect the patient's wishes and reduce stress for loved ones as the disease progresses.

- Adapted intervention strategies

Tailored intervention strategies are personalized approaches designed to meet the specific needs of individuals or groups facing particular difficulties. They are essential in fields such as education, health, social work and psychology. The main aim of these strategies is to offer effective support, taking into account the singularities of each situation, in order to foster the development, well-being and autonomy of the people concerned.

The need to adapt interventions stems from the realization that standardized methods are not always effective for everyone. Each individual has unique characteristics, whether in terms of personal history, culture, abilities or specific challenges. Consequently, a one-size-fits-all approach may not adequately address each individual's needs, and may even be counterproductive. Adapted intervention strategies therefore aim to personalize support, by modifying methods, supports or environments to maximize the chances of success.

In education, for example, teachers are often faced with students with different learning styles, learning disabilities or handicaps. A suitable intervention strategy might involve modifying teaching aids, offering visual materials for visual learners, or using assistive technologies for students with motor or sensory difficulties. In addition, adapting the pace of learning and implementing differentiated teaching can better support students who need more time or extra explanations.

In mental health, professionals must also adapt their interventions to the needs of their patients. For example, in the treatment of depression, some people respond better to cognitive-behavioral therapy, while others benefit more from interpersonal or psychodynamic therapies. Careful assessment of the patient's needs, preferences and history is crucial in choosing the most appropriate therapeutic approach.

Adapted intervention strategies are based on several fundamental principles. Firstly, they require a thorough, holistic assessment of the situation. This assessment enables us to understand the strengths, challenges, resources and needs of the individual or group. It often includes interviews, observations, tests or questionnaires, and may involve different professionals to obtain a complete picture.

Secondly, collaboration is essential. The most effective interventions are often the fruit of teamwork, involving the beneficiary, his or her family, the professionals concerned and, where appropriate, community institutions or organizations. This collaboration ensures that different perspectives are taken into account, and that the strategies put in place are coherent and supported by all the players involved.

Flexibility is also key. Strategies must be able to be adjusted as the situation evolves. It's important to monitor progress regularly, and to be ready to modify the approach if objectives are not being met, or if new challenges emerge. This adaptability ensures that the intervention remains relevant and effective throughout the process.

Another important aspect is respect for personal autonomy and dignity. Intervention strategies must be developed in partnership with beneficiaries, respecting their choices, values and aspirations. This fosters commitment and motivation, essential to the success of the intervention.

Implementing appropriate intervention strategies does, however, present challenges. It may require additional resources, such as time, personnel or specialized equipment. In addition, professionals must be trained to develop skills in assessment, individualized planning and interdisciplinary collaboration. Institutional or systemic constraints can also limit the ability to personalize interventions, notably due to standardized policies or insufficient funding.

Despite these obstacles, the benefits of adapted intervention strategies are numerous. They improve outcomes for individuals, by increasing the effectiveness of interventions and reducing the risk of failure or abandonment. They also contribute to greater satisfaction among beneficiaries and professionals alike, by creating relationships of trust and enhancing the value of each person's skills.

In today's context, marked by a growing diversity of populations and needs, adapted intervention strategies are more relevant than ever. They meet the requirements of inclusion, equity and social justice, ensuring that everyone has access to the support they need to achieve their full potential.

To encourage the development and implementation of these strategies, a number of actions can be taken. The initial and ongoing training of professionals must incorporate skills in individualized assessment, personalized planning and interdisciplinary collaboration. Institutional policies and practices must encourage flexibility and innovation, providing the resources and support needed to adapt interventions.

Research also plays a crucial role, providing evidence on the effectiveness of different approaches and developing new methods to better meet specific needs. Sharing best practices and experiences between professionals and institutions can help disseminate effective strategies and stimulate continuous improvement.

Non-pharmacological approaches

- Reminiscence therapies

Reminiscence therapy is a therapeutic approach that harnesses the power of memories to improve the well-being and quality of life of individuals, particularly the elderly. By delving into past experiences, individuals are encouraged to revisit significant moments in their lives, which can have beneficial effects on their emotional, cognitive and social state. This method is particularly used in the treatment of dementias such as Alzheimer's disease, where it helps to stimulate memory and reinforce a sense of personal identity.

The origins of reminiscence therapy can be traced back to the work of American psychiatrist Robert Butler in the 1960s. Butler observed that elderly people have a natural tendency to evoke their past, a process he termed "reminiscence". He proposed that this inclination is not simply a sign of cognitive decline, but rather an adaptive mechanism enabling individuals to give meaning to their lives and cope with the challenges of aging.

Reminiscence therapy builds on this principle by structuring sessions in which participants are invited to share memories from different periods of their lives. These sessions can be individual or group, and often use stimuli to trigger memories. These may include photographs, music, personal objects, films or even visits to significant places. The aim is to create a safe, stimulating environment where individuals feel comfortable expressing their memories and the emotions associated with them.

The benefits of reminiscence therapy are manifold. Cognitively, it helps to stimulate long-term memory, by strengthening the neuronal connections associated with old memories. It can also have a positive effect on short-term memory, improving concentration and attention. Emotionally, revisiting happy or meaningful moments can bring comfort, boost self-esteem and reduce feelings of depression or anxiety. Participants can experience a sense of accomplishment by sharing their experiences and feeling valued.

On a social level, reminiscence therapy encourages interaction and sharing between participants. In a group setting, it can help break the isolation often felt by the elderly. Exchanging memories creates bonds, sparks discussion and reinforces a sense of community. For families, this therapy also offers an opportunity to better understand the experiences of their loved ones and strengthen intergenerational relations.

Implementing reminiscence therapy requires an empathetic and respectful approach. Therapists or facilitators need to be trained to guide sessions sensitively, encouraging participation without forcing individuals to share memories they prefer to keep to themselves. It's important to create a setting where everyone feels safe to express their emotions, positive or negative, and where sharing is valued.

Ethical considerations are also important. Respecting the privacy and dignity of participants must be a priority. Informed consent is essential, especially in the case of dementia patients who may have impaired decision-making abilities. Therapists must be alert to the potentially negative emotional reactions that certain memories may trigger, and be prepared to offer appropriate support.

Reminiscence therapy can be integrated into a variety of settings, such as long-term care facilities, day centers, hospitals or even patients' own homes. It can be adapted to suit the needs and abilities of participants. For example, for people with severe cognitive impairment, sensory stimuli such as music or smells can be used to evoke memories non-verbally.

Technological advances are also opening up new possibilities for reminiscence therapy. The use of tablets, interactive applications, virtual or augmented reality can create immersive experiences that can enrich sessions. These tools can help overcome certain limitations, such as difficulties with mobility or access to certain stimuli.

- Sensory and cognitive stimulation

Sensory and cognitive stimulation play an essential role in the development and maintenance of brain function throughout life. It involves stimulating the senses and intellectual capacities to strengthen neuronal connections, promote learning, improve memory and contribute to general well-being. Whether for children in the development phase, adults wishing to maintain their cognitive faculties or the elderly facing cognitive decline, sensory and cognitive stimulation offers significant benefits.

The senses are the gateways through which we perceive the world around us. Sight, hearing, touch, smell and taste enable us to interact with our environment, learn and adapt. By stimulating these senses, we activate different regions of the brain, strengthening neural circuits. For example, listening to music can not only bring pleasure, but also improve concentration and memory. Similarly, exposure to a variety of textures through touch can develop tactile perception and motor coordination.

Sensory stimulation is particularly important in children, as it contributes to neurological development. The first years of life are crucial in laying the foundations for cognitive and emotional abilities. Sensory play, such as manipulating objects of different shapes and textures, exploring bright colors or listening to a variety of sounds, promotes awareness and learning. These activities enable children to discover the world, develop their curiosity and build a solid foundation for future learning.

In people with autism spectrum disorders or sensory disabilities, sensory stimulation can help improve communication, socialization and adaptation to the environment. Specific techniques, such as sensory integration, are used to help these individuals process sensory information more effectively, reducing anxiety and maladaptive behaviors.

Cognitive stimulation aims to stimulate higher mental functions such as memory, attention, language, reasoning and problem-solving. It is essential for maintaining and improving intellectual capacities at all ages. Cognitive activities can take many forms, such as board games, puzzles, reading, learning a new language or a musical instrument.

In adults, cognitive stimulation is an effective way of preventing age-related cognitive decline. Studies have shown that people who remain mentally active have a reduced risk of developing neurodegenerative diseases such as Alzheimer's. Participating in intellectually stimulating activities promotes neuroplasticity, i.e. the brain's ability to reorganize itself by creating new neuronal connections.

The combination of sensory and cognitive stimulation can have synergistic effects. For example, art therapy uses artistic media to stimulate the senses and creative expression, while engaging complex cognitive processes. This approach can be particularly beneficial for people with cognitive disorders, improving their communication, self-esteem and quality of life.

In care facilities for the elderly, sensory and cognitive stimulation programs are often set up to support residents. Activities such as gardening, cooking, music therapy or memory workshops are offered to maintain engagement and promote well-being. These programs can reduce depressive symptoms, improve spatial and temporal orientation, and strengthen social ties between residents.

Technology also offers new opportunities for sensory and cognitive stimulation. Mobile applications, adapted video games and virtual reality devices can provide immersive experiences that intensely engage the senses and cognitive functions. For example, virtual reality games can be used for stroke rehabilitation, helping patients to regain motor and cognitive skills.

It's important to tailor stimulation activities to individual needs and preferences. An individualized approach maximizes benefits by taking into account the person's specific abilities, interests and goals. Health professionals, educators and therapists play a key role in assessing needs and setting up appropriate programs.

Moreover, sensory and cognitive stimulation is not restricted to therapeutic or educational contexts. Everyone can integrate stimulating activities into their daily lives to enrich their experience and preserve their mental health. Taking the time to explore new environments, try out new activities or simply pay attention to sensations can have a positive impact on well-being.

- Environmental design to reduce anxiety

Anxiety is a disorder that affects a large number of people, affecting their well-being and quality of life. While there are many causes of anxiety, the environment in which we live plays a crucial role in our emotional state. Thoughtful design of our living and working spaces can make a significant contribution to reducing anxiety levels and fostering a sense of calm and security.

The first aspect to consider is the **organization of space**. A cluttered or disorganized environment can accentuate stress and mental confusion. Decluttering not only clarifies the physical space, but also frees the mind. By sorting objects, discarding or donating those that are no longer useful, we create a more open and soothing space. Adopting effective tidying solutions helps maintain order and facilitates day-to-day management.

Air quality is also essential to well-being. A well-ventilated room reduces the feeling of suffocation and improves concentration. Regularly opening the windows to renew the indoor air is a simple but beneficial habit. What's more, the introduction of houseplants not only helps to purify the air, but also brings a touch of nature that soothes the spirit. Plants such as ivy, sansevaria or ficus are particularly effective at filtering atmospheric pollutants.

Lighting has a major influence on our mood. Natural light is ideal for stimulating the production of serotonin, the happiness hormone. We therefore recommend maximizing daylight by avoiding blocking windows with furniture or thick curtains. In spaces with insufficient natural light, the use of soft-light lamps or fixtures that mimic daylight can create a warm, comforting atmosphere. In the evening, subdued lighting helps prepare the body for rest.

The **colors** used in decorating have a notable psychological impact. Soothing hues such as soft blues, pale greens or neutral tones can reduce nervous system excitement and promote relaxation. Conversely, bright or aggressive colors can increase tension and irritability. Painting walls with serene colors, choosing textiles in soft shades and harmonizing decorative accessories all contribute to creating an environment conducive to calm.

The **acoustics** of the space are another factor not to be overlooked. Surrounding noises, whether from outside or inside, can be a source of agitation. Using absorbent materials such as carpets, thick curtains or acoustic panels can help attenuate unwanted sounds. In addition, incorporating soothing sound elements, such as birdsong, the sound of water or relaxing music, can promote a serene atmosphere.

Smells have an evocative power over our emotions. Aromatherapy uses essential oils to positively influence mood. Diffusing scents such as lavender, chamomile or sandalwood can reduce anxiety and induce a state of relaxation. It's important to choose natural, non-aggressive fragrances, taking care not to overload the air to avoid headaches or allergies.

The ergonomics of the space must also be designed to facilitate movement and daily activities. A functional layout, where everything is in its place and accessible, reduces frustration and stress. For example, arranging furniture so that it can circulate freely, organizing work and rest areas separately, and providing appropriate storage space simplify life and promote well-being.

Incorporating elements of **nature** into the environment is beneficial for calming the mind. Beyond plants, using natural materials such as wood, stone or linen in decorating creates a connection with nature. Images or photographs of landscapes, indoor fountains or aquariums can also add a touch of serenity.

Personalizing space is essential to feeling at one with your surroundings. Surrounding your living space with objects that have personal meaning, such as travel souvenirs, works of art or photographs of loved ones, reinforces your sense of belonging and security. These items evoke positive emotions and can serve as a refuge in times of stress.

Managing **technology** is a contemporary challenge in the quest to reduce anxiety. Electronic devices, while indispensable, can be a source of distraction and information overload. Creating technology-free zones, especially in bedrooms, and establishing moments of disconnection promote mental rest. Setting clear limits on screen use helps prevent anxiety linked to hyperconnectivity.

Finally, it's important to consider the **social influence of** the environment. A welcoming, friendly space encourages positive interaction with others. Organizing the interior to facilitate exchanges, such as arranging seating to encourage conversation, can help reduce feelings of isolation and improve mood.

Managing psychological disorders

- Recognizing depression and anxiety

Depression and anxiety are two common mental disorders affecting millions of people worldwide. Although they may manifest themselves differently in everyone, early recognition is essential for effective management and a significant improvement in quality of life. Understanding their symptoms, their potential causes and how to identify them is crucial to helping sufferers seek professional help and begin the healing process.

Depression is much more than just a temporary feeling of sadness. It is characterized by a persistent depressed mood, a loss of interest or pleasure in activities once enjoyed, and can be accompanied by a variety of physical and emotional symptoms. These include constant fatigue, sleep disturbances, significant weight loss or gain, difficulty concentrating, feelings of worthlessness or excessive guilt, and sometimes recurrent thoughts of death or suicide.

Anxiety, on the other hand, manifests itself as excessive, hard-to-control worry about various aspects of daily life. It can lead to physical symptoms such as palpitations, rapid breathing, trembling, sweating, muscle tension and sleep disturbances. Anxiety can take many forms, including generalized anxiety disorder, specific phobias, panic disorder and obsessive-compulsive disorder.

It's important to note that depression and anxiety can coexist, creating a vicious circle where one amplifies the other. For example, a depressed person may develop anxiety about the future or his or her ability to perform daily tasks, while an anxious person may become depressed due to the mental and physical exhaustion caused by constant worry.

Recognition of these disorders begins with careful observation of changes in behavior, emotions and thoughts. If you or someone you know shows signs such as persistent sadness, disinterest in activities, increased irritability, changes in eating or sleeping habits, it's essential to consider the possibility of depression. Similarly, if excessive worry, panic attacks or avoidance behaviours interfere with daily functioning, anxiety could be the cause.

The causes of depression and anxiety are multifactorial. They can result from a combination of genetic, biological, environmental and psychological factors. A family history of mental disorders, chemical imbalances in the brain, stressful life events such as job loss, relationship breakdown or bereavement can all contribute to their development. So it's important to understand that these disorders are not the result of personal weakness or lack of willpower, but medical conditions requiring professional attention.

The stigma associated with mental disorders can prevent individuals from recognizing their symptoms and seeking help. It is crucial to promote a culture of understanding and support, where talking about mental health is encouraged and normalized. Family and friends can play a key role in this, by offering an attentive ear, expressing their concern in a non-judgmental way, and encouraging the person to seek professional help.

The diagnosis of depression or anxiety must be made by a qualified professional, such as a general practitioner, psychiatrist or psychologist. These experts use specific criteria and assessment tools to determine the presence and severity of the disorder. An accurate diagnosis is essential to develop a suitable treatment plan, which may include psychotherapy, medication, or a combination of both.

Psychotherapy, such as cognitive-behavioral therapy, helps individuals identify and modify negative thought patterns and maladaptive behaviors. It offers strategies for managing symptoms, developing coping skills and improving resilience. Antidepressant or anxiolytic drugs can also be prescribed to correct chemical imbalances in the brain, thereby reducing symptoms and facilitating recovery.

In addition to professional treatment, certain measures can be taken to support the healing process. Maintaining a daily routine, regular physical activity, a balanced diet and adequate sleep all contribute positively to mental health. Relaxation techniques such as meditation, yoga or deep breathing can help reduce stress and anxiety.

It is also beneficial to strengthen social ties by spending time with friends and family, or joining support groups. Sharing experiences with others in similar situations can bring comfort and reduce feelings of isolation.

It's important to recognize that recovery from depression and anxiety is a process that can take time. There may be ups and downs, and it's normal to encounter obstacles along the way. Patience, perseverance and ongoing support are essential to progress towards well-being.

- Communication techniques to soothe the patient

Communication is a fundamental tool in the relationship between caregiver and patient. It is not limited to the exchange of medical information, but also encompasses the emotional, psychological and social dimensions of the individual. Soothing a patient requires an approach that is empathetic, respectful and adapted to his or her specific needs. Effective communication techniques can not only reduce anxiety and fear, but also build trust, improve treatment adherence and contribute to a better care experience.

One of the first steps in calming a patient is to establish warm, caring eye contact. The gaze is a powerful vector of non-verbal communication that can convey compassion and care. By maintaining appropriate eye contact, the caregiver shows that he or she is fully present and attentive to the patient's concerns. This helps build trust from the very first moments of interaction.

Active listening is another essential technique. It involves paying full attention to the patient's words, without interrupting or passing judgment. It also means observing non-verbal cues, such as facial expressions, tone of voice and body language, which may reveal emotions or concerns not expressed verbally. By rephrasing or summarizing what the patient has said, the caregiver demonstrates that he or she has understood his or her concerns, which can help to alleviate anxiety.

Empathy is at the heart of soothing communication. It involves putting oneself in the patient's shoes to understand their feelings and perspectives. By expressing empathy, the caregiver validates the patient's emotions and makes them feel that they are not alone in their experience. Phrases like "I understand how difficult this can be for you" or "It's normal to feel worried in this situation" can bring great comfort.

The choice of words is also crucial. Using language that is clear, simple and adapted to the patient's level of understanding avoids misunderstandings and frustrations. Avoiding medical jargon, or explaining it when necessary, helps patients better grasp information about their health. What's more, using positive, reassuring expressions can help create a more serene environment.

Congruence between verbal and non-verbal communication is important for building trust. Gestures, posture and tone of voice must be consistent with the words spoken. A calm, collected tone, open posture and slow gestures can help reduce patient stress. Conversely, inconsistency between what is said and what is expressed non-verbally can generate confusion or mistrust.

Asking open-ended questions is an effective technique for encouraging patients to express their feelings and concerns. It gives them the opportunity to talk freely about what's on their mind, which can have a cathartic effect. For example, asking "How do you feel about this treatment?" rather than "Do you have any questions?" invites a more detailed and personal response.

It is also essential to respect silences. Moments of pause can allow the patient to reflect and formulate his or her thoughts. Not rushing to fill silences shows that the caregiver is patient and ready to listen to what the patient has to say at his or her own pace.

Humor, used sensitively, can be a way of lightening the mood. It can help reduce tension and establish a more informal connection. However, it's important to get to know the patient well and ensure that the humor is appropriate to the situation and respectful of his or her feelings.

Validating emotions is another technique for calming the patient. By acknowledging and accepting the feelings expressed, the caregiver shows understanding and respect for the patient's emotional experience. For example, saying "I can see you're worried about the operation" legitimizes the patient's feelings and opens the door to further discussion.

Offering clear and precise information about procedures, treatments and expectations can reduce uncertainty and anxiety. When patients understand what's going to happen, they feel more in control of the situation. It's important to check that the patient has understood by asking them to rephrase or by asking comprehension questions.

The caregiver's availability and accessibility also contribute to soothing the patient. By being available to answer questions and taking the necessary time with each patient, the caregiver reinforces the feeling of support and security. Even short interactions can have a significant impact if the patient feels that the caregiver is fully present.

Personalized communication is also important. Every patient is unique, with his or her own experiences, beliefs and preferences. Adapting your approach to take account of these factors shows patients that they are considered as individuals. This can include using their name, respecting their cultural or religious values, and taking into account their communication preferences.

Finally, working with the patient in the decision-making process can increase commitment and reduce anxiety. By involving the patient in the choices concerning his or her treatment, presenting the available options and discussing the benefits and risks, the caregiver encourages a partnership relationship. This gives patients a sense of autonomy and control over their health.

- Collaboration with psychologists and psychiatrists

Collaboration between healthcare professionals is essential to provide comprehensive care tailored to patients' complex needs. Among these collaborations, that with psychologists and psychiatrists is of particular importance, as it enables us to address the mental and emotional dimensions that profoundly influence physical health and general well-being.

Psychologists and psychiatrists play complementary roles in the field of mental health. Psychologists, who specialize in behavioral sciences, focus on psychological assessment, diagnosing mental disorders and implementing non-medication therapies such as cognitive-behavioral therapy. They help patients understand their thoughts, emotions and behaviors, and develop strategies to overcome psychological difficulties.

Psychiatrists, as specialist physicians, are empowered to prescribe psychotropic drugs in addition to providing psychotherapy. Their medical training enables them to understand the complex interactions between physical and mental illnesses, which is crucial for patients with co-morbidities. They play a key role in differential diagnosis, the management of severe symptoms and the medical follow-up of pharmacological treatments.

Collaboration with these professionals enables a holistic approach to the patient. By working together, doctors, nurses, psychologists and psychiatrists can develop integrated care plans that take into account the physical, psychological and social aspects of health. For example, a patient with a chronic illness such as diabetes may also suffer from depression, which affects adherence to treatment. Coordinated care between diabetologist and psychologist can significantly improve clinical outcomes.

This collaboration also promotes continuity of care. Regular exchanges of information between professionals enable consistent monitoring of patient progress. Interdisciplinary meetings, shared records and communication protocols facilitate this coordination. This reduces the risk of redundant interventions, avoids contradictions in the messages conveyed to the patient, and ensures more efficient care.

In addition, working with psychologists and psychiatrists enriches the skills of other healthcare professionals. Nurses and general practitioners can gain a better understanding of psychological distress signals, therapeutic communication techniques and methods for managing crisis situations. This strengthens the ability of the healthcare team to respond to patient needs in an empathetic and effective way.

However, interprofessional collaboration requires a mutual understanding of each other's roles and competencies. It's important to respect specific areas of expertise and recognize professional boundaries. For example, a nurse may identify signs of anxiety in a patient, but refer the patient to a psychologist for further assessment and specialized intervention.

Organizational challenges, such as lack of time, budget constraints or communication difficulties, can hamper collaboration. To overcome them, it is essential to promote a culture of teamwork within healthcare structures. This can include setting up interprofessional training courses, creating spaces for joint discussion and developing clear collaboration protocols.

Confidentiality is another crucial aspect. Information shared between professionals must be treated with the utmost respect for ethical and legal rules. Informed patient consent for the sharing of sensitive information is essential. Transparent communication with the patient about the importance of this collaboration for his or her health can facilitate this process.

Finally, collaboration with psychologists and psychiatrists has a positive impact on patient satisfaction. Feeling listened to and understood in all aspects of one's health strengthens trust in the healthcare team. This can improve adherence to treatment, reduce care-related anxiety and promote a better quality of life.

Thanks

- **To all the dedicated professionals who work with the elderly every day.**

Every day, thousands of professionals devote their time, energy and compassion to serving the elderly. Their commitment goes far beyond mere professional duties; it's a vocation imbued with humanity, patience and respect. These men and women accompany our elders in times of joy as well as hardship, providing support, comfort and dignity to those who have contributed so much to our society.

Their role is essential in a world where the ageing population poses new challenges. They are the pillars that support not only the physical needs of the elderly, but also their aspirations for a life rich in social relationships, meaningful activities and emotional well-being. Whether in care facilities, at home or in communities, these professionals create warm, secure environments that promote autonomy and respect for each individual.

Their work requires a multitude of skills: medical knowledge, interpersonal skills, adaptation to new technologies, understanding of ethical and cultural issues. They demonstrate remarkable resilience in the face of daily challenges, whether managing complex situations, coping with limited resources or navigating constantly evolving healthcare systems.

We owe them a deep debt of gratitude for their tireless dedication. Their contribution is measured not only in terms of the care they provide, but also in the impact they have on the quality of life of the elderly and their families. They are the guardians of human dignity, ensuring that every person can grow old with respect, comfort and joy.

By recognizing their work, we are underlining the importance of supporting these professionals through appropriate training, fair working conditions and a recognition of their role in society. They deserve our respect, support and admiration for everything they do.

To all the dedicated professionals who work with the elderly every day, we offer our sincere thanks. Your commitment makes an invaluable difference in the lives of so many, and your compassion brightens our world.

Table des matières

Préface 13

L'importance de l'endocrinologie et son impact sur la santé globale. 13

Chapitre 1 : Introduction à l'endocrinologie — 15

- Qu'est-ce que l'endocrinologie ? — 15
- Les glandes endocrines et leurs rôles. — 16
- Maladies et affections courantes. — 18
- L'importance du rôle de l'infirmier en endocrinologie. — 20

Chapitre 2 : La réalité quotidienne en service d'endocrinologie — 23

- Structure et organisation du service. — 23
- Interaction avec les patients : les premiers contacts. — 25
- Gestion des urgences endocriniennes. — 26
- Les spécificités du travail de nuit. — 28

Chapitre 3 : Techniques et procédures — 31

- Prélèvements sanguins et tests hormonaux. — 31
- Administration des traitements. — 33
- La prévention des complications. — 35
- L'éducation thérapeutique du patient. — 37

Chapitre 4 : Pathologies et prises en charge — 39

- Le diabète sucré : une épidémie mondiale. — 39
- Les troubles de la thyroïde. — 44
- Les affections des glandes surrénales, hypophyse et parathyroïdes. — 51

Chapitre 5 : Communication et collaboration — 54

- Communiquer efficacement avec les patients et leur famille. — 54

- La gestion des cas complexes : coordination avec d'autres services.   55

Chapitre 6 : L'endocrinologie pédiatrique   58

- Les défis spécifiques des enfants et adolescents.   58
- Transition de l'endocrinologie pédiatrique à l'endocrinologie adulte.   60
- Collaboration avec les familles pour une prise en charge optimale.   61
- Pathologies endocriniennes spécifiques à la pédiatrie.   64

Chapitre 7 : Endocrinologie et grossesse   66

- Gestion du diabète gestationnel.   66
- Troubles thyroïdiens pendant la grossesse.   68
- L'importance du suivi endocrinien pré-conceptionnel.   70
- Accompagnement post-partum et allaitement.   72

Chapitre 8 : Endocrinologie gériatrique   75

- Les changements endocriniens avec l'âge.   75
- Gestion des maladies endocriniennes chez le patient âgé.   77
- Importance de la polypharmacie et des interactions médicamenteuses.   79
- Soutien à la qualité de vie et à l'autonomie.   82

Chapitre 9 : Technologies et télémédecine en endocrinologie   85

- L'utilisation des pompes à insuline et des moniteurs continus de glucose. — 85
- Consultations à distance et suivi virtuel des patients. — 87
- L'importance de la formation technologique pour les infirmiers. — 89
- La télémédecine comme outil de collaboration interdisciplinaire. — 91

Chapitre 10 : Aspects psychosociaux en endocrinologie — 94

- Comprendre les impacts émotionnels des maladies endocriniennes. — 94
- Accompagnement psychologique spécifique : dépression, anxiété, troubles de l'image corporelle. — 95
- Soutien aux groupes spécifiques : adolescents, personnes transgenres, patients infertiles. — 97
- Techniques de communication pour aborder des sujets sensibles. — 99

Chapitre 11 : Nutrition et endocrinologie — 102

- Principes de base de la nutrition en endocrinologie. — 102
- Diététique spécifique : Diabète, troubles thyroïdiens, obésité. — 103
- Collaboration avec les nutritionnistes/diététiciens. — 105
- Éducation du patient à l'autogestion alimentaire. — 107

Chapitre 12 : Endocrinologie et sport — 109

- Gestion du diabète chez le sportif. — 109

- Importance des hormones dans la performance sportive. ... 111
- Accompagnement de l'athlète endocrinien. ... 112
- Prévention des troubles de l'endocrinologie liés au sport. ... 115

Chapitre 13 : L'endocrinologie dans différentes cultures ... 118

- Approche interculturelle en endocrinologie. ... 118
- Gestion des croyances et des pratiques traditionnelles. ... 120
- Sensibilisation aux besoins spécifiques des différentes populations. ... 122
- Adaptation des soins selon le contexte culturel. ... 124

Chapitre 14 : Pharmacologie en endocrinologie ... 127

- Médicaments couramment utilisés et leur mécanisme d'action. ... 127
- Interactions médicamenteuses à surveiller. ... 129
- Importance de l'adhésion au traitement. ... 130
- Effets secondaires courants et leur gestion. ... 132

Chapitre 15 : Approche holistique en endocrinologie ... 135

- L'importance de l'équilibre entre le corps, l'esprit et l'âme. ... 135
- Techniques complémentaires : méditation, yoga, acupuncture. ... 136
- L'importance d'une approche centrée sur le patient. ... 138
- Collaboration avec des professionnels alternatifs ou complémentaires. ... 140

Chapitre 16 : Enjeux de la santé mondiale en endocrinologie — 143

- Épidémiologie des troubles endocriniens à travers le monde. — 143
- Défis et opportunités dans les pays à ressources limitées. — 145
- Collaboration internationale et programmes d'échange. — 146
- L'endocrinologie face aux crises mondiales : pandémies, changements climatiques. — 148

Chapitre 17 : Santé numérique et endocrinologie — 151

- Les applications mobiles pour le suivi et l'éducation des patients. — 151
- Utilisation des objets connectés (wearables) pour le suivi en temps réel. — 153
- Les plateformes de gestion des données patients. — 155
- L'importance de la cybersécurité en santé. — 157

Chapitre 18 : Prévention en endocrinologie — 160

- Promotion des habitudes de vie saines. — 160
- Vaccination et prévention des maladies endocriniennes. — 162
- Rôle éducatif de l'infirmier en prévention. — 163
- Collaboration avec d'autres professionnels de la santé en prévention. — 166

Chapitre 19 : Endocrinologie et chirurgie — 169

- Préparation du patient pour les interventions chirurgicales. — 169
- Soins post-opératoires en endocrinologie. — 171

- Collaboration avec l'équipe chirurgicale. — 173
- La réhabilitation et le retour à la normale. — 174

Chapitre 20 : L'endocrinologie et les autres spécialités médicales — 177

- Collaboration avec la cardiologie. — 177
- Interaction avec la néphrologie. — 179
- Relations avec la gynécologie et l'andrologie. — 180
- Interface avec la psychiatrie et la psychologie. — 182

Chapitre 21 : Gestion des situations difficiles et conflictuelles — 185

- Gérer les conflits avec les patients et leur famille. — 185
- Collaboration dans un environnement parfois tendu. — 187
- Naviguer dans les situations émotionnellement chargées. — 189
- Ressources et soutien pour les infirmiers en situation difficile. — 191

Chapitre 22 : L'avenir de la formation en endocrinologie — 194

- Évolutions pédagogiques et formats de formation. — 194
- La place de la simulation en formation. — 195
- L'autoformation et les nouvelles technologies. — 197
- L'importance des retours d'expérience et de la formation continue. — 199

Chapitre 23 : Perspectives d'avenir et innovations — 201

- L'évolution du rôle de l'infirmier en endocrinologie. 201
- Les nouvelles technologies et leur impact. 203
- La recherche clinique : une opportunité pour les infirmiers. 205

Conclusion 207

- L'importance du dévouement, de l'empathie et de la compétence dans le soin des patients endocriniens. 207
- Glossaire des termes médicaux. 209
- Ressources pour une formation continue. 213
- Bibliographie pour approfondissement. 216

www.ingramcontent.com/pod-product-compliance
Lightning Source LLC
Chambersburg PA
CBHW071651240526
45469CB00021B/1939